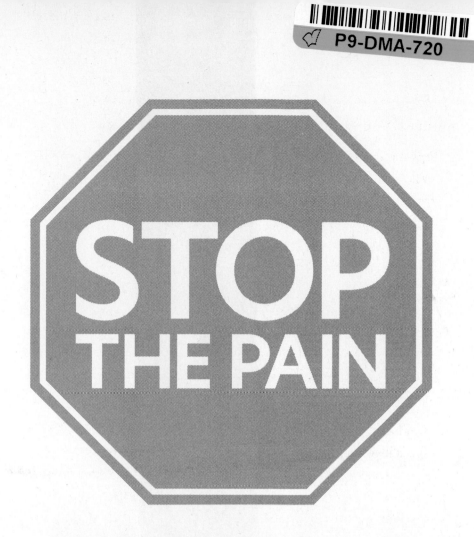

STOP THE PAIN

THE SIX TO FIX

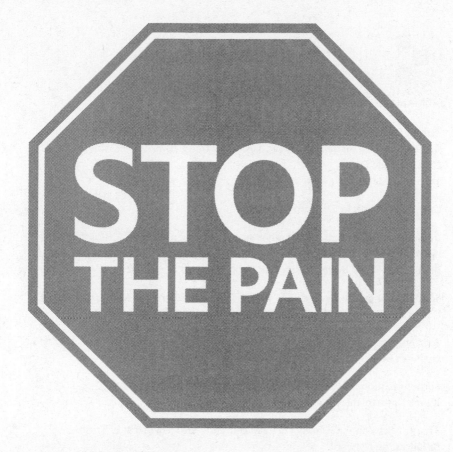

THE SIX TO FIX

Dr. Scott K. Hannen

Trilogy Publishing Group

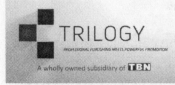

Trilogy Christian Publishers
A Wholly Owned Subsidiary of Trinity Broadcasting Network
2442 Michelle Drive
Tustin, CA 92780

10 9 8 7 6 5 4 3 2 1

Library of Congress Cataloging-in-Publication Data is available.

ISBN 978-1-64088-904-0
ISBN 978-1-64088-905-7 (e-Book)

Dedication

This book is dedicated to my son Chas who continues to stand and live by the faith and grace of Jesus Christ. Chas is an inspiration to whoever hears his story. He has overcome pulmonary atresia from birth, seizures during high school, and most recently Hodgkin's Lymphoma during his college years. While writing this book I watched him fight the good fight of faith, overcoming this horrible disease, which caused me to be inspired to write this book through one of the hardest struggles in my life. The strength behind this book was birthed through my son's ability to never give up and to stand when I know he felt like falling. Through his strong faith and determination, he is living proof of God's faithfulness.

He is stronger and healthier now than he has ever been in his entire life. I praise God for my son and look forward to seeing him step into his calling with great expectation. We will bless and support him as he continues to be an inspiration to encourage those who are facing life-threatening challenges. If Chas can do it, so can you! His courage and determination were the conformation I needed in order to have the confidence to step out into reaching the entire world with this message. Chas, you are and will always be my best buddy! I love you, son.

Acknowledgments

I want to thank my wife for standing with me in agreement as we go through life's challenges. She has been such a blessing to me through this time of writing the book you hold in your hand. I commend and appreciate her and her efforts including the many hats she has had to wear in order to take pressure off of me so I could focus on writing this book. Aneesa, you are the love of my life!

I want to give a special thanks for my GTH family whose loving faith and support have been overwhelming. Only God could bring together such an amazing group of people. It's such an honor to be called their pastor. GTH, you are the best sheep in the world!

I certainly want to extend my gratitude to my nephew Dr. Mitch and the clinic staff who spend many days treating and taking care of my patients so I am able to dedicate the time necessary to bring this message to the world.

I cannot forget to thank Bobby, Travis, Barry, and Dwaine, my four lifelong best friends. What would I do without you guys in my life? Thanks for always being there for me.

I want to thank my TBN family for your continued support and especially Matt and Laurie Crouch. Matt, thank you for being the big brother I never had. You've taught me so much about so much. Laurie, thank you and the boys for always treating me like family. You guys are the best.

Finally, I want to thank my family for always believing in me and especially my precious mother whom I have never had a cross word with throughout my entire adult life. She has always been my greatest supporter and biggest fan. Mom, I love you more than I will ever be able to express.

Table of Contents

SECTION 1
Biomechanics

CHAPTER 1: **The Need for Change**

CHAPTER 2: **Biomechanics**

CHAPTER 3: **Detect and Correct Spinal Misalignments**

CHAPTER 4: **The Core of Support**

Immune Response

CHAPTER 8: **Immune Responses**

Foreword

Dr. Scott has been taking care of our family's health needs for decades now.

My father had quite a collection of canes later in his life because of a knee injury he had years prior. Scott treated his knee over a single weekend while in Orlando and Dad never had to use a cane again! There was no use of drugs and no surgery. Years of suffering and pain were gone for the rest of his life just by helping to restore the proper function to his knee. So, Scott has our attention when he talks health.

Laurie and I were at lunch with Scott recently, riveted as he unpacked the miraculous — some might say the "medically impossible" — supernatural healing of his son Chas, who had been suffering life-threatening Hodgkin's Lymphoma.

It's a powerful, real-life testimony that could have ended very differently. I can only imagine what it would be like to have a life-threatening disease assigned to your only child. Scott briefly shared with us how overwhelming that threat can be, especially when you try to handle it from a day-to-day, "let's just try and get through this" mentality.

As we were wrapping lunch together, Laurie leaned in and asked what turned out to be a life-altering question, "Scott, what was it that you feel you learned the most from this experience?"

He didn't need to think about the question very long; "Laurie, God taught me something. I've learned that faith doesn't speak to the present, it speaks to your future, and your future speaks to your present."

After I about spit my ice tea across the table, I wanted to make sure I'd heard him right and asked him to repeat his answer: "Faith doesn't speak to the present, it speaks to your future, and your future speaks to your present," he said a second time, but this time with even more conviction.

Scott continued, "I was believing for my son to be healed, but that was having 'hope' and not living by faith. That's when the revelation came to me that his healing was in the future — and that's where I needed to go, to the finished work of Christ. And that reality needed to speak to my present situation.

"That was the catalyst that enabled me to get over my fear and frustration. Faith was speaking to our future and our future spoke to our present, and the future we saw is now a reality. My beloved son is completely free from cancer!"

If there ever were one, this became one of life's "Aha Moments" for Laurie and me!

There's a profoundly important revelation in what Scott proclaimed that day about the very nature of faith, and we've reflected on it often — and not just in the context of physical healing and seeing yourself well before you are.

For example, I recently found a typewritten note folded up in my dad's Bible from his then-assistant, dated July 10, 1973. He'd apparently kept it for decades as a reminder of God's faithfulness. It impacted me so much I immediately posted it on my Instagram feed.

It read, "Unless the Lord performs a miracle, we will not have a payday on Friday. We are in the red $371.64. I have held the following checks..." and she goes on to list them. "PS: July 11's deposit (will be) $246.63."

One thing I can tell you categorically about my father is that he was a man of extraordinary faith. I watched him walk it out day by day, miracle by miracle. And by faith, his "future" was the only thing that could possibly "speak to his present" shortfall in the strained startup days of this first, struggling station in southern California, a shower curtain serving as the "studio" backdrop.

But despite struggling with average deposits of just a few hundred dollars at the time, well short of what they needed to even make payroll, imagine if he'd been able to fast forward into his future and see what TBN would become...

Imagine if at that moment Dad could have seen TBN one day covering the entire globe as the world's largest and most watched faith-and-family broadcaster, reaching over 175 nations across the earth with inspirational and engaging programming 24 hours a day in 14 languages and on 32 global networks proclaiming the hope and grace found only in Jesus.

Can you imagine how quickly the stress and anxiety of such a moment would dissipate? I can't know for sure, but Dad may have well done just that—and after lifting it up to the Father, perhaps he had every assurance that TBN's present financial "sickness" was temporary at best.

In any circumstance that requires faith, if we look to our future in Christ and lay our burdens on Him, we can virtually eliminate fear and uncertainty. And it's that "future that speaks to our present" in life-altering ways. Then, when we have our faith destination clearly in sight, our present "GPS" so to speak takes over, faithfully guiding us turn by turn.

We all know Hebrews 11:1 KJV says, "Now faith is the substance of things hoped for, the evidence of things not seen." But sometimes it's easy for us to confuse "faith" with "hope." It's not. Rather, I've come to understand faith is the substance of things hoped for.

In other words, it's real. It's substantive. And it's in your future, not your present circumstance. This (Scott's) revelation about faith reminds me of when my late friend, Kim Clement, often used to quip, "You're somewhere in the future and you look much better than you look right now!"

As it relates to physical healing, doctors nearly universally agree there is a strong faith/spiritual component that they can't chart and diagram in medical school. People of strong and abiding faith, like Chas and his folks, Scott and Aneesa, often experience results that defy the natural. We authentic "People of the Way" do so because we've accepted the finished work of the cross and receive the words, "by His stripes we are healed."

It's like something is stitched into our DNA once we're walking by faith and not by sight.

When people are dealing with debilitating pain and suffering, it's easy to get stuck in the right now and with the awfulness that accompanies it. The revelation that Christ put help and recovery in your future is the wisdom that can speak to your present so that your faith can operate from a different viewpoint.

So, the idea that you can "stop the pain" from a spiritual perspective is yet another "amazing grace" provision, set aside for authentic followers of Jesus. But there's another key component: We are physical beings while on this earth and, because of that, there are real-world things that are required of us as well — things we must actively be willing to do in our proactive partnership with our Creator/Healer.

"We are what we eat!"

Admittedly, this is an overused axiom we hear most of our life, yet one we tend to treat with reckless *abandonment* until we're in serious trouble. However, when we are in pain and illness, we're suddenly eager to learn about what our role is to begin to heal.

"We are what we think" is probably a more appropriate way to approach our road to recovery because clearly our choices can make the difference.

Over nearly two decades of friendship, I've learned from my very studied, [physician] friend, Scott, that virtually all disease starts *(from the choices we make, good or bad)* [in the gut]. [Would be that we would do what's right for our bodies ("temples") sooner, but if ever the proverbial "gut check" is in order, it's when we're experiencing pain.]

The fact that we can largely reset our *body systems* [gut] in just a *few weeks and months* [30 days] is in itself a miraculous provision of our Creator. But even that takes a bit of proactive "doing" on our part, as you'll better understand in the coming pages.

Our spiritual and physical partnership with God is an awesome thing to think about, and one we should take seriously. It's the age-old principle that "We do what we can, and God will do what we can't."

It's like the old fisherman's proverb that we need to "keep both our faith and works oars in the water" and in equal measure. Pulling with only one or the other will have us going in circles, getting nowhere fast.

The book you're fortunate enough to be holding in your hands explores both God's part in healing these very complex bodies that are "fearfully and wonderfully made," and our part in properly understanding the vital role we play in stopping the pain.

It's our prayer from this day forward that you begin to enjoy a whole new understanding of faith and your abundant, pain-free life!

Matt & Laurie Crouch
Trinity Broadcasting Network

BIOMECHANICS

CHAPTER ONE

The Need for Change
The Road to Recovery

I've often heard it said, "From the hardest struggles come the greatest gifts." This has certainly been the case in my own life. My son was recently diagnosed with Hodgkin's Lymphoma, a potentially life-threatening type of lymphatic cancer. There's no way you can prepare yourself for the shock when that diagnosis is pronounced over your only child and it hits your understanding just what that means.

I have been in clinical practice for nearly thirty years and have treated people from around the world including very high profile individuals. Many of those people have had similar life-threatening conditions. Yet there is a new and different realization when it shows up in your household. For more than a year now we've been battling this horrific disease, standing in the faith of God while also using the best possible scientific advancements for cure that are available. Just a few weeks ago, while finishing the last part of this book, our greatest gift was awarded. Our son, Chas, is one hundred percent cancer free and is stronger and healthier than he has been in his entire lifetime.

Sometimes it seems like life isn't fair. Chas is a fine young man whose Christian morals and values are even an inspiration to me. There's no father who wouldn't continue to brag about the integrity of his son, and I am no exception. Chas had earned a full scholarship by winning challenge matches that placed him as the number one seed on his college tennis team. He was also the captain of his team and maintained a 4.0 grade point average through the process. He was finishing his pre-med classes so he could enroll in medical (osteopathic) school and "suddenly" a lump showed up on his neck. After an initial exam, CT scan, and biopsy, the doctors at the University of Alabama Birmingham hospital diagnosed him with Hodgkin's Lymphoma. "Boom!" A sucker punch straight to the gut.

Chas was doing everything that was expected of him and even more. He was the model son and in most areas an overachiever, and "suddenly," all of that was seemingly about to be stripped away. It would have been easy for Chas to fall into self-pity and crumble under the pressure, but instead he chose to rise up and fight. My son should be an inspiration to all who read this book.

There are many of you who are facing similar struggles, whether it be with cancer or any other type of sickness, disease or disorder. Don't allow your present circumstances to determine your future outcome—rise up and fight! I want to encourage you in the Lord as He has encouraged my family. "Through the hardest struggles come the greatest gifts." There's no better reward for the hardship we endured than the gift of my son's healing. It was through this struggle I was challenged to find the time and resources to write this book so others could also experience their breakthrough. Through the hardest struggle in my life I was given the gift that you hold in your hand: *STOP THE PAIN*. My prayer is that the gift given to me through my family's struggle can be a gift to you and your family. Perhaps it can be a lifeline so that you will be able to celebrate your victory when your battle comes to an end. Thank you for allowing me to share this gift, my life's work, with you. From the bottom of my heart I wish you the best and hope you enjoy this book.

God's Plan for Your Body

You should not have to live with pain, suffering, disorders, or disease. There's no reason to just accept a diagnosis that has no cure and continue to do nothing about it. God made you a body that heals itself! It just has to be given what it needs. You cannot expect it to do a job if it does not have the right tools. However, if you give the body everything it needs to do its job, I am thoroughly convinced that there is almost nothing that it can't cure. There are always other options that can scientifically and systemically bring possible correction. You have to ask the right questions in order to get the correct answers.

This book is in no way designed to offer false hope or empty promises. It is certainly not a replacement for good medical care. This book is for anyone who has been suffering with pain and can't find solutions from what they are currently doing. This information is intended to provide understanding that causes us to ask questions that need to be answered and hopefully provides a lot of those answers. Perhaps after reading this you may be able to provide your physicians with other insights that offer them more clues in order to help them solve your issue. Physicians have hundreds of patients to keep up with. You only have to keep up with you. No one knows you better than you. This information is being provided to train and equip you to be able to look into your situation and circumstances, and help to sort out the things necessary to bring a better quality of health to your life. The more you understand about how your body works, the more informed choices you can make in order to bring about correction. It is my greatest hope that after you complete this book you will be able to find the assistance you need to take the steps necessary to enable you to STOP THE PAIN.

Beware of Frauds

There are so many medical fads that are out there right now. That is why I do not like people to search on the Internet and try to get advice about their health problems. The Internet is full of people who sell things. The marketing experts sell everything as the latest and greatest thing. It's amazing how convincing some of these marketing ploys can be. They offer pseudoscience mixed in with hype and cause confusion for those who are not adequately educated in the subject matter. There is no panacea, no magic bullet, no super pill or potion. People ask me on a continuous basis, "What should I take so I can feel better?" My answer is always the same, "Whatever your body needs to fix the problem." Most people try to find answers out of desperation and as a result they become victims of these mass marketers. Many of these sales pitches are promoted by fraudulent claims and even are endorsed by individuals who pose as physicians. Beware of those who add to their names titles like "NMD," "nutritional expert," and "doctor," but they do not list their credentials.

Another tactic that is used is the term "health coach." All of these questionable titles are used by people who mislead the public into thinking they are as qualified as a physician who has been through years of training and clinical proficiency testing so that the public at large can trust them. That is what a licensed physician is—a board-certified caregiver who is required to stay current in their specialty. If someone makes a specific recommendation for someone about their health and is not licensed to do so, it is against the law and that person is charged with practicing medicine without a license. These frauds are driven by their own egos and greed, and usually play on people who are desperate, appealing to their desire to seek relief, and take advantage of them monetarily. The reason for years of training, testing, and proving proficiency is so the consumer is safe from these snake oil salesmen and have reliable and qualified physicians to consult for their health needs. When you start searching for help, especially in the arena of natural health, it is buyer beware!

The only licensed primary health care providers in all fifty states are medical physicians, osteopathic physicians, and chiropractic physicians. Medicare and most major insurance companies will cover the cost of care by licensed physicians. There are certain naturopathic physicians, doctors of acupuncture, and Oriental medical doctors who went to accredited schools who are licensed in a few states and they are proficient and legally qualified as well.

Many of the people who display those fraudulent titles have received mail order or online degrees and are not qualified licensed practitioners. This is such a disappointment for those who have gone through the necessary process to be properly trained and licensed. Make sure, before you receive any health advice from anyone, that you see the credentials of the one who is giving that advice and make sure they are valid.

Product fraud is another problem that the consumer needs to be aware of. Make sure when you choose a product that it passes three quick inspections:

1. The content of the main desired ingredient in the product is the actual active form that can be absorbed without being destroyed by the digestive system so it can bring the desired benefit.

2. The active ingredient matches the effective dose that is being recommended by scientific clinical studies and is not a diluted version. Often marketers put negligible amounts of certain popular ingredients in order to include them on the label so they can use them in their advertisements.

3. Make sure the company does regular batch testing on their products to evaluate for ingredient content and potency.

Three Questions for Those Who Need Relief

Everyone who needs relief or cure from sickness, pain, crises, or anything debilitating or uncomfortable should ask themselves three life-changing questions to help them to take steps toward their road to recovery.

1) **Where have I been?** i.e.- What have I been doing right, what have I been doing wrong? Are there unhealthy habits I've developed? What lifestyle have I adapted?

2) **Where am I right now?** i.e.- Am I doing better or worse than usual? Am I willing and prepared to do whatever it takes to bring the desired changes into my life?

3) **Where do I want to be?** i.e.- How do I want to see myself in the future? What goals am I prepared to set for myself and commit to in order to promote the lasting change that needs to happen in my life?

The first thing that needs to happen before anyone can change is the self-realization that change is needed. The next thing is an honest self-evaluation in order to develop a winning strategy that will accomplish the change. These important questions are paramount and essential for preparing for a lifestyle change. Use this book as a tool to help you to better understand why you or those you care about are suffering from sickness and pain.

The Bible says the principal thing we must gain is wisdom. It's kind of like trying to solve a riddle. It can seem almost impossible to solve until someone tells you the answer. Suddenly, the nearly impossible seems so simple to solve. Hopefully this book will give you answers that can solve many of the health riddles that you've been challenged with. The information presented has been collected from shared clinical research, referenced material, and years of clinical experience and collected clinical "pearls" that have been the result of personal self-discovery. It's my greatest hope that as you explore the material listed in this book, that your own self-discovery will lead you down the road to recovery and will equip you with the tools you need to finally STOP THE PAIN once and for all.

> **The first thing that needs to happen before anyone can change is the self-realization that change is needed.**

CHAPTER TWO

Biomechanics

The Purpose of Pain

The one main cause that drives people to go to see the physician, to make a lifestyle change in their life, or to motivate them to do most anything is a sensation we are all well acquainted with called **pain**. Pain is important because it is a primary motivator to take action; however, there are mechanisms and causes that underlie the pain you experience in your body throughout your life that you should be aware of.

Pain is nothing more than a symptom, but it is amazing how it can get your attention. People have pain for different reasons; it is experienced in many different ways. Some people have painful joints. Some people have painful muscles. For some people pain makes them feel sluggish, stealing their energy and causing them to feel run down. Still others have different pain thresholds. Certain ones can tolerate high levels of pain stimulation and experience very little pain. Yet others may have the slightest irritations and as a result have seemingly debilitating pain. For some, doing moderate activities may cause them to build up acids and other by-products in the system making them stiff and sore, which can quickly lead to pain. Others can endure excessively high levels of physical and emotional stresses and have no symptoms at all. The pain possibilities are endless. The take-away message is that we are all uniquely different, and in order to get to the bottom of solving our chronic pain issues, the focus needs to be on detecting and correcting the things that are specific to our individual needs.

Some people have pain from their emotions and their feelings. Some people have torment in their minds and their thoughts because of the painful things that happened in their life. Whatever the reason, emotional or physical pain can produce a lot of chemical changes in the body. These changes can produce some pretty dramatic effects in the body, especially those that cause different types of pain. The very fact that someone is experiencing pain indicates that something is out of balance. The real questions are "What caused it to be out of balance?" and "What can be done to bring that back into balance?" This book is focused primarily on what causes physical pain and how to correct it.

There is an epidemic of pain that's producing a generation that's trying to find relief in a bottle. The problem is these medications are highly addictive and are proven to cause problems of their own. These pain-relieving drugs, particularly opioid drugs, stimulate the pleasure centers in the brain so powerfully that according to clinical studies it only takes five days to become addicted. That can be a real problem considering the average prescription is given for seven days.

Substances, including prescribed drugs, are rated on the amount of pleasure they produce in the brain on a scale called the "Brain Pleasure Rating System." Some of the most highly addictive foods score around two hundred. Sex scores around two hundred and sixty on the scale. Let's face it, food and/or pornography are extremely difficult temptations to resist for the average person and as a result, there are millions of people who become addicted because of the intense pleasure these can produce in the brain. When you start dealing with pain medications like opioid drugs, the stimulation jumps up into a whole different league. The pleasure rating for low-level opioids scores around seven hundred and for methamphetamines around fifteen hundred. Perhaps realizing what these numbers represent can demonstrate what the state of mind is for someone using these "prescription drugs." This hopefully explains why so many normal, responsible people who have high integrity, and are of good moral character, can still fall prey to this powerful addiction. Experts say the United States is in the throes of an opioid epidemic, as more than two million Americans have become dependent on or abused prescription pain pills and street drugs. During 2017, there were more than 72,000 overdose deaths in the United States, including 49,068 that involved an opioid, according to a provisional CDC count. More than 130 people died every day from opioid-related drug overdoses in 2016 and 2017,

❝ ...the opioid crises is not a 'drug' problem. It's a 'pain' problem.' ❞

according to the US Department of Health & Human Services (HHS). The number of opioid prescriptions dispensed by doctors steadily increased from 112 million prescriptions in 1992 to a peak of 282 million in 2012, according to the market research firm IMS Health.

Let's face it: something needs to change and it needs to start now. First, we need to recognize the opioid crises is not a "drug" problem. It's a "pain" problem. The word "addiction" is derived from a Latin term for "enslaved by" or "bound to." Anyone who has struggled to overcome an addiction — or has tried to help someone else to do so — understands why. Addiction exerts a long and powerful influence on the brain that manifests in three distinct ways: craving for the object of addiction, loss of control over its use, and continuing involvement with it despite adverse consequences.[1] Additionally, the intensified dopamine response in the brain that mood-altering drugs produce does not naturally stop once the behavior is initiated or completed (as is the case with natural reward behaviors such as eating or having sex); as a result, cravings for the rewards associated with the drug continue to occur, even during drug use, which leads to compulsive, repetitive use.[2] And while overcoming an addiction is possible, the journey is often a long and painful one. Most people who initially become addicted to prescription drugs are not searching for pleasure, they are trying to find relief from pain, so pain is the problem. This book is my contribution to trying to establish more natural non-addictive approaches to eliminate pain.

If this crisis is ever going to end, we all have to change the way we approach the treatment of chronic pain and suffering. I feel the best place to start is by going to the root of the problem. The best treatment for this epidemic is prevention. Let's look at some basic fundamental principles about how the body operates and continue to progress until hopefully, by the end of the book, you will have the tools to understand where pain comes from, how and why it progresses, and most importantly how to eliminate it. This book is a tool that you can use in order to help you STOP THE PAIN..

Pain is simply the body reporting when something is out of balance, something is out of alignment, something is not right, is not in its proper homeostasis; when this happens the body will report to the brain, "Hey, something is wrong!" Next, the brain perceives the pain and attempts to get the body to do something or not to do something in response. For example, if the foot is traumatized, the foot reports the damage to the brain, the brain sends a pain response and the perception is, "Ouch!" If the foot is traumatized and hurting, do you really think you should be walking on it? Obviously not! The brain understands this concept and says, "You are not walking on it." If you try to walk on it, you will experience pain in an attempt to keep you from injuring it further. If you can understand this simple concept, that this mechanism is operating in your body every time you have pain, that your brain is trying to stop the body from hurting itself, or it is trying to report to you that there is something wrong, then you are already miles ahead of what the mainstream concept of pain is.

Most of us have been involved in the personal treatment of pain. In the day and age in which we live, we often try to cover up the pain. The pain clinics try to manage pain. It is even called "pain management." Why would someone want to manage the system that is reporting to the brain that something is wrong? Why would anyone want to manage this built-in alarm system and attempt to make it go away and never address the underlying cause? The truth is, that is exactly what is going on right now when it comes to pain and suffering.

Most everyone takes over-the-counter medicines, NSAIDs (non-steroidal anti-inflammatory drugs), aspirin, and acetaminophen at some time or another. These drugs are designed to disrupt the reporting system, to dismantle the pain warning signs, and conveniently cover up the problem.

Have you ever been driving down the road in your car and notice one of those dash lights come on? Why is that light coming on? Let us say it is the oil light. It is warning you that something is wrong. Likewise, that is what pain does. It sends a warning that something is not right. Now you can take a piece of black tape, stick it over that dash light, and the warning will disappear. However, you must ask yourself, "Is that really a smart maneuver?" That is exactly what is happening when you reach for one of those over-the-counter medications. It is just like putting tape over the warning sign. Sometimes a little bit of perspective goes a long way.

Chronic pain

Pain is often the first warning sign from the body letting us know that something is wrong. That's why no one should ever ignore pain or try to cover it up with medication without first establishing the cause. Most chronic pain is treated with pharmacological measures, including acetaminophen and NAIDs such as ibuprofen, naproxen, and the newer cyclooxygenase-2 inhibitors. Acetaminophen is generally effective in managing mild to moderate pain, but its chronic use has long been associated with potential liver toxicity, which can be fatal, even in therapeutic doses.[3] Nonsteroidal anti-inflammatory drugs are commonly associated with gastrointestinal and renal side effects and, consequently, their use is inadvisable for many individuals.[4] Muscle relaxants generally are not prescribed for chronic use because of their sedating effects and, like acetaminophen, generally are more effective for mild to moderate pain.[5] Antidepressants, such as amitriptyline, have long been prescribed for the management of pain, and especially for the generalized pain of fibromyalgia, but they generally produce only a modest, transient benefit and significant side effects.[6] Opioid-based pain medications do provide temporary relief; however, besides producing relatively common gastrointestinal side effects, opioid analgesics may produce physical and psychological dependence, so that many doctors and patients are uncomfortable with their use for chronic, nonmalignant pain.[7] Consequently, the search continues for novel ways to control chronic pain.

Pain may be unpleasant but it sure does do a good job of getting our attention when something is wrong. When pain becomes a menace is when it becomes chronic, meaning it persists over a long time. Nerve endings become very efficient at expressing pain. Like a body builder continually stimulating the muscles by repetitive activity, chronic pain fibers also are enhanced when they are continually and repetitively stimulated. This type of pain can be very difficult to treat with conventional methods. These fibers form networks that release certain chemicals that promote pain and discomfort. The longer someone has the pain the more established the network of pain becomes. The only way to STOP THE PAIN is to break this chronic pain cycle.

I remember one my patients (whom I will refer to as Tina to protect her true identity).

Tina walked into my office complaining of chronic pain that had recently started getting worse to the point she was having trouble managing it throughout her body. She also was having trouble sleeping at night because she couldn't get comfortable due to the pain. She had tried medication, massage, pain management, acupuncture, and had even been adjusted by a chiropractor. These treatments gave her a little temporary relief, but the pain quickly returned in every case. After taking her case history I decided to order some blood work.

Upon reviewing the result, I was quickly drawn to a significant deficiency in her vitamin D levels. I immediately gave her a clinical dose to continue taking for several weeks. The most amazing part of this story is that after about two weeks she had absolutely no pain in her body. She couldn't believe it. Her life was completely back to order in a very short time. Sometimes pain that seems so complicated can be solved in a very short time by something as simple as a vitamin deficiency. I want to encourage you by letting you know that it doesn't matter how long you've had the pain, how bad it is, or even what type of pain it is, if you are willing to think outside the box, your solution could be just one simple step away. If you have pain there is a reason for that pain. The key is not to stop looking until you find that reason.

I had another patient we will refer to as Carla. She came into my office complaining of severe headaches that were debilitating. She stated that she had had them for several years but over the last year she had been under a lot of stress and the headaches had gotten worse. The headaches were getting so bad that she couldn't focus on her schoolwork and as a result she had to drop out of college. Carla had been to a variety of medical doctors to include an ear-nose-throat specialist. They prescribed her medications but they made her feel spacey and didn't seem to help the pain. She decided not to take them. She resorted to taking some over-the-counter headache medications along with some aspirin. These took the edge off but never resolved the pain.

After completing her examination, I decided to take some upper cervical x-rays.

When I pulled the films up on the computer screen I immediately saw what I felt the problem was. I explained to her that the first vertebra in her neck was severely misaligned and was putting a significant amount of pressure on the nerves in that area and also was restricting some of the blood flow at the base of her skull. After treating her using an upper cervical technique called *Atlas Orthogonality* (meaning "the quality of being at right angles"), her headaches disappeared immediately and have not returned for several years. Once again the problem was detected and corrected and we were able to STOP THE PAIN and keep it from recurring.

Still another patient came into my office complaining of chronic neck, shoulder, and back pain. He said in the morning his hands would ache and his shoulders would throb with pain. He had been to several physicians who had tried steroids, antibiotics, muscle relaxers, anti-inflammatory drugs, and pain pills. He had absolutely no relief. The last doctor he saw before coming to see me prescribed Prozac and told him the reason he was in pain was because he was depressed. You can imagine how he felt after trying all of these approaches yet having no success.

While examining him I noticed some soreness around the maxillary sinuses and on each side of the nose. I treated him for a sinus problem using a technique in which swabs are dipped in a silver protein solution, inserted in the sinuses, followed by a nasal specific release maneuver opening up the turbinates that drain into the back of the throat. He experienced immediate relief. Tears began to roll down his cheeks as he explained to me that it was the first time in years that he had no pain in his body. That's right. The cause of his neck, shoulder, and back pain was coming from his sinuses.

Many times I find that the pain people are experiencing doesn't originate in the same area they experience the pain. Pain can be present for a lot of reasons.

Oh My Aching Joints

When you wake up in the morning, does it take you a little while to get going? Do you feel stiff and sore in your muscles or around your joints? When you clench your fists or bend your knees, are the joints tight, sore, or even painful? When you walk up and down steps, or bend over, do you have to take your time because of the discomfort you experience in your back and body? Do sudden movements cause you to have excessive pain? Millions of people around the world experience some form of arthritic, traumatic, or chronic pain and look for relief in a potion or lotion, hoping it will give them results. Musculoskeletal (MSK) pain is common worldwide. In economically developed countries such as the United States, between 14 percent and 26 percent of the adult population suffers from chronic pain or arthritis,[8] approximately 11 percent report chronic, widespread pain,[9] and MSK disorders account for 15 percent of work-loss days.[10]

The fact is, arthritis, tendinitis, bursitis, fasciitis, and all of the "itis" gang have many causes and multiple mechanisms that initiate and promote its presentation. The worst thing someone can do is to just ignore the symptoms or take something to cover them up while the problem rages on. Symptoms are there as a warning. Don't ignore them, instead investigate the reason behind them. When it comes to dealing with symptoms, the five most dangerous words are "maybe it will go away." On the flip side, pain is often one of the last symptoms someone may experience when they have an underlying problem and one of the first symptoms to disappear when receiving treatment. It is a necessary warning sign but it does not indicate the status of a health condition. A good example of this is when someone has a severe disease such as cancer. That person may not be experiencing any pain at all, yet go in for a routine yearly physical and the physician may diagnose cancer because of abnormal lab results. As a matter of fact, when a physician is palpating a lump or a bump to determine whether it's malignant or not, the consistency of hard, fixed, nodular, and usually non-painful lumps are the diagnostic parameters that are used to identify it as a cancerous lesion. Normal health is not the mere absence of

> **Normal health is not the mere absence of symptoms.**

symptoms. When someone treats the pain instead of the cause they are ignoring a warning allowing the underlying problem to progress without detection.

Let's look into this thing called pain, where it comes from, why it is there, and what we can do to fix the underlying causes that initiate it. This book is divided into **six main sections**. Each of these sections explains in great detail to help you better understand cause of pain. There are also **six recovery protocols** that provide the instruction on nutrients, recommendations, and explanations on how to bring correction to these areas. **Six to fix, six ways to fix it!** There are varieties of people who will read this book, from people who hold PhDs, to people who may not have finished grade school. If there are parts that seem a little too "doctorish," please keep reading because there will also be a simple explanation there as well. This style of writing is intentional so that other physicians as well as patients can read the information on the level they need to receive it. **Each section has words in bold type for better emphases, clarity, and understanding.** This also makes it easier when you want to go back and review the primary points. There is a quick review at the end of each section with a list of **pain stoppers** taken from each section. This makes compliance much easier and allows you to quickly access the steps without having to reread the entire section. The study of pain can be a very complicated and intricate endeavor. It's taken me more than thirty years, hundreds of thousands of dollars, and years of education and board certifications, along with nearly thirty years of clinical hands-on experience to narrow it down to the six things to fix in order to STOP THE PAIN. I am honored to be able to share what I have learned with you.

1. How addiction hijacks the brain; Harvard mental newsletter: Published: July, 2011

2. Wise, R. A. (1996). Addictive drugs and brain stimulation reward. Neuroscience, 19, 319-340.

3. Larson AM, Polson J, Fontana RJ, et. al. Acute Liver Failure Study Group Acetaminophen-induced acute liver failure: Results of a United States multicenter, prospective study. Hepatology. 2005;42:1364–72. [PubMed] Bolesta S, Haber SL. Hepatotoxicity associated with chronic acetaminophen administration in patients without risk factors. Ann Pharmacother. 2002;36:331–3. [PubMed]

4. Henry D. Assessing the benefits and risks of drugs. The example of NSAIDs. Aust Fam Physician. 1990;19:385–7. [PubMed].

5. Tofferi JK, Jackson JL, O'Malley PG. Treatment of fibromyalgia with cyclobenzaprine: A meta-analysis. Arthritis Rheum. 2004;51:9–13. [PubMed] Childers MK, Borenstein D, Brown RL, et. al. Low-dose cyclobenzaprine versus combination therapy with ibuprofen for acute neck or back pain with muscle spasm: A randomized trial. Curr Med Res Opin. 2005;21:1485–93. [PubMed].

6. Carette S, Bell MJ, Reynolds WJ, et. al. Comparison of amitriptyline, cyclobenzaprine, and placebo in the treatment of fibromyalgia: a randomized, double-blind clinical trial. Arthritis Rheum. 1994;37:32–40. [PubMed].

7. Moulin DE. Opioid analgesics for chronic nonmalignant pain. Can J CME. 1996;2:137–43.

8. Lawrence RC, Hochberg MC, Kelsey JL, et. al. Estimates of prevalence of selected arthritic and musculoskeletal diseases in the United States. J Rheumatol. 1989;16:427–41. [PubMed] Magni G, Marchetti M, Moreschi C, Merskey H, Luchini SR. Chronic musculoskeletal pain and depressive symptoms in the National Health and Nutrition Examination. I. Epidemiologic follow-up study. Pain. 1993;53:163–8. [PubMed].

9. Croft P, Rigby AS, Boswell R, Schollum J, Silman A. The prevalence of chronic widespread pain in the general population. J Rheumatol. 1993;20:710–3. [PubMed].

10. Felts W, Yelin E. The economic impact of the rheumatic diseases in the United States. J Rheumatol. 1989;16:867–84. [PubMed].

CHAPTER THREE

Detect and Correct Spinal Misalignments

Oh My Aching Back

Low back pain is the second most common physical complaint among Americans, exceeded only by headaches. Many people complain of having neck pain and mid-back, pain as well. The first thing you need to understand when you are dealing with any type of back pain is that the back consists of one spine. We divide it up into neck, upper back, mid back and low back, etc., for the sake of discussion and identifying the level of pain, but the fact is it is one spine and functions as one unit. When the vertebrae in the spine get misaligned, it causes a biomechanical dysfunction called a **spinal subluxation**. The definition of a spinal subluxation is "the condition of a vertebrae that has lost its proper juxtaposition with the one above or the one below, or both; to an extent less than a luxation; which impinges nerves and interferes with the transmission of mental impulses." This medical mouthful basically means the bones in the spine are not in the correct alignment where they should be. This misalignment disrupts the nervous system causing abnormal signals to be sent to the brain affecting balance, coordination, and function.

The same spinal tracts that become disrupted as a result of the subluxation are also involved in maintaining and balancing organs, systems, and body processes. Spinal subluxations not only produce pain, but also produce dysfunction and imbalances in the body systems and processes as well. The most common problems caused by subluxation are pain syndromes. These can range from basic neck and back pain, to chronic aching pain and soreness, to severe and debilitating pain. There are so many health conditions people experience that may be corrected by using chiropractic treatment to realign the spine. For example, someone may have a spinal subluxation that's causing high blood pressure. Still another person may have one that is causing them to have indigestion or even constipation. Still yet another has one that's causing vertigo or migraine headaches. Typically, no one would think that a spinal subluxation could cause these issues, but the truth is chiropractors have been making these corrections for more than a hundred years. The only health professionals trained and licensed to detect and correct spinal subluxations are chiropractic physicians. Chiropractic is no longer considered to be some esoteric type of practice, but over the last many years is proven as a valid form of treatment confirmed by evidence-based medicine. This is quite obvious considering chiropractic physicians are licensed by all fifty states and recognized by the federal government as primary health

> **The only health professionals trained and licensed to detect and correct spinal subluxations are chiropractic physicians.**

care physicians. That's fact, not opinion.

Subluxations have often been referred to as "the silent killer" because if they go undetected they can cause chronic imbalance and dysfunction that can lead to conditions that literally drain the life out of you. Correcting them can improve anything from eliminating pain to restoring normal body functions and processes. Making these corrections allow patients to experience health at an optimal level, naturally providing them with other options besides the use of pharmaceutical drugs.

Where's the Pain Coming From?

Often when people experience pain in a particular place in their body, the problem originates from somewhere else besides that area. Countless people have walked into chiropractic clinics with pain in their low back. The doctor detects and corrects a problem in the neck, and the low back pain immediately resolves. The same can occur in reverse order where a problem detected and corrected in the low back resolves neck pain. How can this be possible? The answer is quite simple, but the explanation can be quite lengthy and highly complex. However, a basic understanding will suffice when someone needs to find help for this problem.

The bones in our skeletons are hooked together with strong ligaments. Between the bones is a soft tissue shock absorber called cartilage that is very resistant to wear and tear and keeps our bones from jamming into each other as we engage in activity. There are small fluid-filled discs in between the bones in the spine that serve as shock absorbers so the spine can be flexible. Muscles attach to the bones so they can move and function in a variety of positions. These muscles also help to stabilize the bone structure and assist in protecting and facilitating its function. Muscles in the spine help to support the skeletal posture and allow us to be flexible and to maneuver in multiple ranges of motion.

Our musculoskeletal systems are comprised of a complex system of levers, pulleys, and a variety of articulating surfaces. Biomechanically these systems all work together to allow us to be able to move and function at our optimal ability. When these systems are well maintained and in proper balance and alignment, they are very efficient, and with the appropriate training can offer us a high level of agility, mobility, strength, and support. However, when these systems become imbalanced or weakened, they can create a host of problems that cause abnormal binding and grinding, wear and tear, inflammation and irritation, pain and strain, lack of mobility and agility, instability, and even disability.

These conditions are usually diagnosed as **musculoskeletal conditions** (such as arthritis, tendinitis, bursitis, ligament sprain, muscle strain, myofascial, etc.). Most all of these conditions are associated with significant pain and, if left untreated, can progress into chronic conditions that leave their victims helpless and hopeless living in constant pain.

The majority of people have experienced one or more of these conditions at some point in their lives. I would go as far as to say that most people wake up in the morning and have some form of stiffness, soreness, or even pain most every day. How many times have you been riding in your car and your neck and shoulder muscles tighten up and get sore? How about the strain you feel on your lower back when you bend over or try to tie your shoes? Do you get headaches? Do you have sore spots on your body or in your joints? Do you experience nerve pain or numbness and tingling in your extremities? These are just a few of the complaints that people live with. Many who suffer like this think their pain is caused by stress.

Some write it off as the aging process. Still others have turned to medications that merely cover up the symptoms instead of correcting the problem. Stress may exacerbate an existing condition or even speed up its progression, but very rarely is it a primary cause of someone's problem. Musculoskeletal tissues do degenerate respectfully with the aging process, and although it may affect our strength, endurance, mobility, and agility, in and of itself should not produce pain. Pain is not a "normal" condition. It is a normal response that warns us of an underlying problem, much like an alarm system.

> **Pain is not a 'normal' condition. It is a normal response that warns us of an underlying problem, much like an alarm system.**

One analogy I like to use when explaining how the spine can cause pain is a **"twisted dishrag."** If I twist a dishrag at both ends, my hands will draw closer together. Why? Twisting (torsion) causes **compression**. When spines get twisted, they compress tissues and in some cases even the nerves get pinched. This causes abnormal stimulation that the body may interpret as pain and can cause dysfunction or even loss of function. If this is the cause of your pain, then taking pills or changing your diet is probably not going to correct the problem. There's on old saying, "You can't eat your way out of a biomechanical problem any more than you can adjust your way out of a nutritional deficiency." The obvious solution would be to remove the torsion through some type of manual treatment such as chiropractic, osteopathic, physical therapy, or soft tissue manipulation.

Addressing the cause of pain allows you to choose the exact treatment tool that you need to bring complete healing. People ask me on a regular basis, "What do you think I should take for my pain?" My reply is always the same. "It depends on what the cause of the pain is." Pain is one subject in which everyone should get educated.

There are some conditions that you can make general recommendations for, and they will respond well. However, most people have problems that were created by their particular lifestyles and habits; therefore, the treatment protocol should be tailored to fit each person based on their specific needs. This is the approach that gets the best results. One good example of this would be if someone presented into the clinic with arthritis accompanied by significant joint pain from the chronic inflammation. They may visit a chiropractor who detects and corrects their spinal subluxations and because the biomechanics improve so much by reducing the excessive stress on the joints, the joint pain and inflammation may completely resolve. This particular case did not need anti-inflammatory drugs or cortisone injections. The spinal subluxations were the cause of this particular problem and that is why the problem resolved when they were removed. The next patient who walks into the clinic may have the exact same signs and symptoms as the previous arthritic patient, but after correcting the spinal subluxations that patient may not feel any relief. This is because that was not the cause of that particular arthritic condition. The same diagnosis can often have entirely different treatments. Different problems require different solutions. There's no magic bullet. There's not one cure for pain. The best way to find and fix a pain problem is to treat the person and not the condition. This information is provided in order to give more options in resolving the causes of pain and not

> **"The best way to find and fix a pain problem is to treat the person and not the condition."**

merely trying to relieve it.

The majority of people who suffer from pain due to biomechanical problems have suffered some type of trauma. Motor vehicle accidents, slips and falls, blunt force traumas, sports injuries, recreational accidents, and falling off the monkey bars at school are just a few examples of how people injure their musculoskeletal system. Then of course there are more subtle ways such as bumping your head on the way into the car, raising up and hitting your head on the cabinet, playing weekend warrior and overdoing it, and even sleeping on your stomach or maybe with your neck and back in a twisted position.

If you constantly drive on streets with cracks, bumps, and potholes, the front end of your car may shift out of proper alignment, causing uneven wear and tear (degeneration) on your tires and resulting in an uncomfortable ride. The same thing happens with our bodies. We seem to be constantly doing things that cause our spines to get misaligned and our joints and soft tissues to sustain injuries. When these structures shift out of their proper alignment they cause abnormal wear and tear on the joints causing degeneration. From chronic, repetitive poor posture, all the way to acute traumas, we continue to assault our bodies with typically no realization of what's really taking place when it's happening. Most of us think when the pain and soreness subside from an injury, we are okay. However, the majority of the time structures heal in a posture that's been compromised and is biomechanically disadvantaged. That means the next time that person tries to lift or strain, their leverage system has been altered and transfers weight in an irregular fashion. This creates a biomechanical disadvantage and puts too much stress on the wrong structures, usually resulting in an injury. The majority of my patients who present with back pain weren't lifting transmissions or motor blocks when they caused their problem. They usually injure themselves bending over to tie their shoe or reaching for the tooth-paste. You might ask, "How can you throw your back out reaching for the toothpaste?" The answer is simple. The body was already biomechanically disadvantaged when they reached to get it. When your biomechanics are compromised, even the simplest of tasks can leave you vulnerable to injury.

It's quite common in people who don't get their musculoskeletal systems evaluated for imbalances to develop chronic muscle and joint pain. When imbalances sustain over months and years the tissues literally change their shape as well as lose optimum func-tionality. For example, it's quite common to see the heels on people's shoes worn down more on one side than the other. This should ob-viously indicate that person's gait has been altered from normal and is displacing more weight on one of the shoes than the other. There's a term called **plastic deformation** that describes what happens to the soft tissue structures when tissues are compressed or stretched continually for long periods of time. The soft tissues actually change their shape. Those tissues that are compressed get shorter and those that are stretched get longer. This is usually caused from musculo-skeletal imbalance from traumatic events. When weight is distrib-uted more to one side than the other, the musculoskeletal system is compromised, causing tissues to become compressed and joints to become misaligned. Sometimes a simple chiropractic adjustment can correct misalignment and put the body back in the center.

Quite often, however, the adjustments will not stabilize and have to continually be repeated. This is because the soft tissue has to be addressed as well. When tissues are compressed for any length of time they constrict and can literally choke out nerve and blood flow. The compressed tissues need stretched back out and the stretched tissues need to have the strain alleviated. These tissues need to be rehabilitated through physical therapy, deep tissue massage, myofascial stripping, trigger point therapies, exercise, stretching, and other modalities that help decompress and remove abnormal strain from the muscles and soft tissue structures.

Let's return to the example of the misaligned front end on your car. Why should you get it realigned? You do that because if you don't there will be uneven wear and tear on the tires and will cause them to wear out prematurely. When you realign the front end the tires no longer suffer from the additional wear and tear. This is how it works with spinal and joint biomechanics. When structures get misaligned they begin to suffer from the additional wear and tear (like the tires). When referencing the body the term for wear and tear is **degeneration**. When joints are misaligned from subluxation and from the soft tissues being under constant strain, they degenerate causing inflammation and pain. **Degenerative joint disease** is a common cause for pain and suffering. Relieving the biomechanical stresses from the joints can bring dramatic and in many cases complete relief from this type of pain and suffering. Of course there are other factors associated, but for the sake of this discussion, the biomechanics play a significant role.

There are multiple things we do in the course of our day that can cause our bodies to be biomechanically disadvantaged. One common cause of back pain is sitting in a recliner or propping the head up on the back of the couch while lying down. This causes an unhealthy traction on the neck and spinal structures causing spinal cord tethering. Low back pain and headaches usually follow soon after this occurs. People who sleep on their stomach will almost always have neck or back pain. The reason is when lying face down, the head has to twist to the side to breathe. When someone stays in the position that causes the neck to be twisted for a few minutes up to a few hours, they can expect neck and back pain. In many cases, it can produce headaches as well. The elderly often use canes causing them to lean forward and have to tilt the head upward causing neck tension, pain, and balance problems. The cane should be adjusted up to its full height or else they should use a walking stick so their posture can be upright alleviating the postural stress.

There have been many times when patients have presented with neck, back, shoulder, arm, leg pain or even headaches that are caused by poor quality mattresses or pillows. In many cases they are just old, worn out, and need to be replaced. If someone has no pain when they go to bed but wake up in the morning and has it, there is a high probability that it is time to update the sleeping surfaces. Pillows are the cheapest so swap those out first. When shopping for a mattress, get one that has at least 1000 coil springs or more so it doesn't create worn-out spots and cause the sleeping surface to become unlevel. A good practice is to flip and rotate your mattress every couple of months. This prevents the formation of worn-out spots and divots.

One of the most common ways people misalign their pelvic structures is by crossing their legs. When the legs cross, the pelvis has to shift itself to accommodate the new position. This position places binding pressure on the hip and sacroiliac (SI) joints. The joints get locked in that position and can no longer support the weight as efficiently because the range of motion has been impaired causing binding and grinding in the joints. This can be quite painful and make you move around as if you had aged thirty years. Most people have no idea this even exists and they just think they slept on it wrong or perhaps write it off as old age. The next thing to expect is knee pain because at the other end of the leg bone that goes into the hip is the knee. The majority of the knee pain eliminated at my clinic is corrected from the pelvis, and the knee itself never has to be addressed. Sometimes it is as simple as correcting a pelvic misalignment and the knee pain completely resolves and the mobility returns to normal. Propping the leg up while sitting in the chair can cause the same problem. If you spend a lot of time at a desk or computer, set the screen at eye level so your neck isn't strained by looking down constantly. Simply lowering the chair or raising the screen can accomplish this. If you are tired of living in pain, dealing with soreness and stiffness, and are fed up with taking pills to cover up the symptoms, it would probably be a really good idea to get yourself checked out by a chiropractor so your body's biomechanics can be aligned back to normal. People regularly maintain their homes, vehicles, and lawns, yet forget to regularly check the spinal and joint biomechanics that make enjoying life possible. Regular chiropractic checkups should be a no-brainer for anyone who wants to STOP THE PAIN.

CHAPTER FOUR

The Core of Support

Core Muscles

The only way the low back and spine can provide and maintain proper shunt stability for the body is to have strong core muscles. **Shunt stability** is the ability for your body to stabilize in one area so it can leverage another. This is what allows us to lift, move, and carry objects. Think of your core as a strong column that links the upper body and lower body together. Having a solid core creates a foundation for all activities. The problem is the majority of people stop doing three important things once they reach the age of around thirty: **sprinting**, **spinning**, and **jumping**. These maneuvers fall into a category called plyometrics (jump training). These, combined with short burst explosive movements, help improve maximal performance. These are awesome exercises to build agility, flexibility, and mobility. However, never attempt plyometrics until first you strengthen your core muscles or you may injure yourself because of lack of stabilization. Most people think that the way you protect the back from injury is to strengthen the back muscles. That may be of some benefit, but actually the correct way to accomplish this is to strengthen the core muscles. The torso powers all of our movements. The abdominals and back work together to support the spine when we sit, stand, bend over, pick things up, exercise and more. Your core muscles are the muscles deep within the abdominals and back, attaching to the spine or pelvis. Some of these muscles include the **transversus abdominis**, the muscles of the pelvic floor, and the oblique muscles. Another muscle that is involved in moving the trunk is the **multifidus**. This is a deep back muscle that runs along the spine. It works together with the **transversus abdominis** to increase spine stability and protect against back injury or strain during movement or normal posture. The **psoas** muscles are also extremely important for providing deep spinal support especially involving motions combined with leg movements.

Proper "core strengthening" techniques can support the combined function of these muscle groups. When the core muscles are strong they make the entire biomechanical system more resistant to injury. There's no way to tell how many patients that I've had who started doing their core exercises faithfully and their spinal pain, aches, and body pains completely disappeared. Even patients who had constant recurring pain syndromes stabilized as a result of staying consistent in doing these exercises. In my opinion, one of the safest and simplest ways to improve pain in the body is to strengthen the core muscles and maintain them on a consistent and regular basis.

Listed here are four simple exercises (**Four for the Core**) that I have recommended for almost thirty years that have helped stabilize the core muscles of my patients. Start the exercises at 5 repetitions (reps) per each one progressive, without stopping until all four are completed for 1 set. Wait for 1 minute and repeat again and then again for a total of 3 sets. Slowly work up to 25 reps for each exercise for a total of 3 sets. When you reach that level of intensity the core should be strong. Continue to maintain that level doing the exercises at a minimum of 3 times per week.

Four for the Core:

1: MODIFIED ABDOMINAL CRUNCH

- Lie down on the floor on your back and bend your knees.
- Place your arms across your chest.
- Bend forward as if you were doing a sit-up but only come up about 8-12 inches.
- Then return back but don't let your shoulders rest on the floor after starting. This keeps constant tension on the abdominal muscles.
- Repeat these until the desired amount is completed.

2: BENT KNEE MODIFIED ABDOMINAL CRUNCH

- Repeat the same technique as the last exercise except this time lift both feet off of the ground about 1-2 inches through the entire set.

3. SKY WALKERS

- Lie flat on your back.
- March like a toy soldier with the arms and legs locked stiff and straight. Point toes toward ceiling on both sides. The heels cannot touch the ground once you start the exercise. This keeps constant tension on the core muscles through the entire exercise.
- The leg that is raised should be straight with the bottom of the foot and the heel pointed to the ceiling when it reaches the top.
- The other foot should remain about six inches off of the ground with the foot pointed upward.
  (To incorporate the psoas muscle the foot can be turned out when raising the leg).
- Do the desired amount of reps and then relax.

4: HEELS TO THE HEAVENS

- Lie down flat on your back.
- Point the bottom of your heels toward the ceiling with your legs straight but not locked at the knees, this is starting position.
- Start with left heel and push it toward the ceiling about six to eight inches while both feet remain in the air and return to starting position.

- Next, push both heels to the ceiling and return to starting position.
- Then push the right heel to the ceiling and return to starting position.
- Finally push both heels to the ceiling again and return it to starting position.
- That completes one repetition.
- Do the desired amount of reps and relax.

Stretching

Tight muscles can cause anything from lack of motion, pain, stiffness, and soreness, to neck pain, back pain, extremity pain, TMJ dysfunction, and headaches. The possibilities are endless. Muscles affect the way we do life. There is a covering around each muscle called the myofascia and sometimes that tissue gets tight. It's kind of like when you put a cotton sock in the dryer for too long. When you put it on, it squeezes your foot. That's what happens when the fascia gets too tight around the muscles. It restricts movement and blood supply and causes the muscle to experience tightness, aching, burning, and discomfort. In many cases the fascia gets injured from the chronic pulling or trauma and it inflames. If anyone has ever had burning, or sharp pain in the heel or arch of the foot this is probably what's wrong. This particular condition is known as **plantar fasciitis**. The pain can be intense and even debilitating at times. Most physicians treat this condition with cortisone injections and anti-inflammatory drugs. These do usually provide relief but the condition usually returns in a very short period of time. Why? The cause of the problem has not been addressed.

For **plantar fasciitis**, one popular idea is to stretch the calf muscle to relieve the heel pain. The problem with this approach is that it is further stressing an area that's already injured and inflamed. If someone had an inflamed area anywhere else in the body they wouldn't even consider stretching it. Then why consider stretching an inflamed heel? Believe it or not, the correct way to treat it is to stretch the **anterior leg muscles** and not the posterior (the exact opposite). The correct stretch is to point the toe down plantar flexing the foot. One easy way to do it is to flatten the top of the foot by pointing the toe down and sitting on the foot that has the inflamed heel. Slowly continue stretching it until the pain is reduced. The second stretch is to do a **figure four stretch** in a seated position pushing the knee towards the floor. The stretches should be done on both sides. If some-

> **Research clearly shows, cold muscles don't stretch.**

one has a one-sided problem anywhere in the body and has not had a localized trauma involved, then it's more than likely caused from something shifting off from center alignment. These types of problems are usually easily detected and corrected by chiropractic care. When someone has myofascial tightness and restrictions, the muscles should first be warmed up by light exercise before stretching them. If not, research clearly shows, cold muscles don't stretch. Therefore warming them up, then slowly and passively stretching the muscles, while moving the muscle in the direction actively while applying the stretch, will bring the most benefit. This holds true for almost every muscle. People who suffer with tendonitis anywhere in their body almost always have a muscular imbalance, misalignment, or a postural shift that's not being addressed.

There are many other types of core exercises as well as beneficial stretches you can do to bring flexibility and stability to your musculoskeletal system. These are just a few that I've recommended to my patients over the years that are usually quite effective. Get started with these and if you want to branch out and try some others that would be fine, but always remember that if you feel pain during an exercise, don't do it. I'm not talking about the discomfort that's present because it's been a while since you've exercised or even if your muscles burn a little from fatigue. I'm referring to actual "pain." The last thing you want to do is injure yourself while you are in the process of improving your performance.

FIX#1: Pain Stoppers

○ Stay out of recliners.

○ Don't prop your head on the back of the couch or chair.

○ Get a new pillow.

● Rotate your mattress and check to see if you need a new one.

○ Stop crossing your legs.

○ Sit at eye level with your computer by lowering the chair or raising the screen.

Do **Four for the Core** exercises at least 3 times weekly (possibly try adding some plyometrics after a few weeks).

Stretch tight muscles after warming them up and actively move them in the direction of the stretch.

Get regular adjustments to maintain proper alignment from your chiropractic physician. Osteopaths who perform manipulations, physical therapists, and licensed massage therapists can also be of great benefit, especially when it comes to soft tissue problems like muscular and myofascial issues.

OXIDATION

Stop the Oxidation

Replenish and Restore the Antioxidant System

One common question that people ask consistently is, "What is disease?" They want to know what sickness is. How do we name it? Where does it come from? In order to answer these questions we have to go to the cells. When the rate of cell damage exceeds the rate of repair, that is sickness. In other words, you are damaging faster than you are healing. When that is prolonged, the sickness turns into disease — 'dis-ease' — over a period of time. If you have damaged cells in your heart and it goes on prolonged, it is diagnosed as heart disease. If there are damaged cells in the liver, it is called liver disease; if it is in the colon — colon disease. Wherever the cell damage is, a disease process is developing in that area and the disease or the disorder will be

> **When the rate of cell damage exceeds the rate of repair, that is sickness.**

named based on the location.

Sometimes disease is named after the scientist who discovers the damaged cells and how they were damaged. **Parkinson's disease** is a good example of this naming process. The disease is named after the English doctor **James Parkinson**, who published the first detailed description in *An Essay on the Shaking Palsy* in 1817. Another way diseases get their names is when someone of celebrity status gets diagnosed with a strange disease. **Lou Gehrig's Disease** is a good example of this. **Henry Louis Gehrig**, nicknamed "**the Iron Horse**," was an American baseball first baseman who played his entire professional career (17 seasons) in Major League Baseball for the New York Yankees, from 1923 until 1939. Lou Gehrig was one of the most popular baseball players of all time. He was diagnosed with an incurable neuromuscular disorder and was forced to retire at age thirty-six and finally passed away two years later. It was a rapidly progressing disease of the neurological system called **amyotrophic lateral sclerosis**. The disease literally folds people up and puts them into severe spasms and contractions while wasting them away to nothing. So the famous athlete Lou Gehrig made the disease well known and now it is commonly referred to as **Lou Gehrig's Disease**.

There are many different ways diseases are named, but the focus is on understanding the mechanism that starts the process of disease through cellular damage.

Oxidation and Inflammation

Science is designed to quantify and qualify information. Scientific data is compiled from research studies, double-blind studies, comparative data, laboratory findings, clinical research, and especially from experience working with patients day in and day out, and practitioners comparing notes to see what works and what does not.

It is amazing when all this information is compiled together the amount of clarity it can bring if interpreted correctly. It is a great way to get rid of some of the fallacies that are out there about what is effective and what is not. It is so ironic that taking information from one person is called plagiarism. Taking information from a lot of people is called research. Research clearly shows that there are two primary mechanisms that cause cellular destruction in your body. These two mechanisms wreak havoc on the cells in the system causing an array of dysfunction, diseases, and disorders. They are **oxidation** and **inflammation**. These two processes can have devastating effects on your overall health if not kept under control by the body processes. Everything in the body starts with the cell. Cells multiply and combine to produce tissues, organs, and all of the masses of your body. Everything is made up of cells. If something is damaging those cells, then it is probably contributing to sickness or disease.

> **...taking information from one person is called plagiarism. Taking information from a lot of people is called research.**

We know about cellular damage and understand that is the underlying cause to disease. It would make sense that there would be a way to stop, or at least to slow down, that damaging process. For example, when the brain cells (the neurons) are damaged over a period of time, there is associated inflammation. Any time something becomes damaged, it starts to inflame because the response to injury is inflammation. Have you ever rolled your ankle? You sprain the ankle; you damage the tissues; what happens to the ankle? It swells. Well, lets say, in the brain you have damaged neurons from oxidation, inflammation, chemicals, trauma, and other things that cause damage to neurons. The brain begins to inflame, swell. When something has been swollen for a long period of time, it also causes more cell damage, so it is a vicious cycle. Inflammation in the brain caused from cells being damaged can have a significant effect on the way we experience life.

One of the most significant processes that causes damage to the cells is oxidation. This, in turn, causes inflammation that creates this chronic damaging effect in the body. Every time you eat you have to convert food to energy. During this process oxidation is a by-product. Every time you breathe in air, it is not a good form of oxygen; it has to be converted in the body to usable oxygen. During the process of that conversion, the by-product leftover is oxidation. Every time you exercise, there are by-products left over in those conversions that produce oxidation. You can eat over-cooked foods or hydrogenated oils that also cause it. You can ingest certain chemicals or be exposed to them, and they can cause oxidation in the system. You can acquire certain microorganisms that produce cell damage in your body by stimulating immune responses that will cause oxidation. All of these things create oxidation.

What is oxidation? Oxidation is simply a destructive process that damages cells. Have you ever cut up apples for a snack? You slice them just right. You lay them on the tray and they look so nice and fresh. You go into another room for fifteen or twenty minutes to do something else and when you come back, something awful has happened to the apples. The apples are brown. Is that a good change or a bad change? That is a bad change. The longer they sit, the longer they oxidize. The longer they oxidize, the more they break down, the more they degenerate, and the browner they turn as a result. You can see it in front of your eyes. That is what oxidation does to the cells in your body.

Have ever left a shiny piece of metal outside for a few days exposed to the elements? What happens to that metal if you leave it out in the weather? Rust! Rust is another word for the degenerative effect of oxidation. Is that a good change or a bad change? It is a bad change. It breaks down and tears down the metal over a period of time. You can see it with your eyes. This is another example of how oxidation damages the cells throughout the body causing sickness and disease.

If you have ever seen paint on a car that has been out in the sun for prolonged periods of time, it starts to fade. The paint loses its luster because the paint oxidizes. Is that a good change or bad change? It is a bad change. Oxidation accelerates the aging process and damages cells in a way that causes them to age at a more rapid rate.

After understanding the way oxidation damages the body, it is clear that we need a strategy to stop this from happening. However, there is another problem, because we have to eat, we have to breathe, and we should be exercising. Every time we do, we create oxidation. So what is a person to do? How do we get around this? Remember, if you leave oxidation for a long period of time, it damages cells. This, in turn, produces inflammation. Right? When you chronically inflame and it stays inflamed for a long time, what does it do to cells? It damages them. Now the vicious cycle begins, **too much oxidation = too much inflammation, too much inflammation = too much cell damage, too much cell damage = more oxidation and inflammation…and the cycle continues**.

Do you see why when some people get sick they say, "I have been fine my whole life, and all of a sudden, all of this stuff starts happening to me. I was fine. I had been doing great until_____, and now it's out of control and getting worse. It keeps coming in waves and layers." Have you had conversations with people and heard this same story? Perhaps you have seen a loved one go through this process and watched them go downhill in a very short period of time, from perfect health to sickness and disease, just like that. They go to the doctors who diagnose it as this condition or that condition, give it this name or that name, yet the person continues to get worse. Who cares what you call it? Naming the condition based on the areas that are damaged so a medication can be prescribed to cover those symptoms to help them cope with the pain is not the solution. Symptom-based treatment may be necessary as a first step or even as an adjunctive measure to assist with the pain until the true problem is dealt with, but it does not solve the problem. (The information in this book is in no way attempting to disgrace, undermine, or even criticize current medical practices. This information is being provided to attempt to provide a new way to look at the causes of pain so more effective corrective types of care can be recommended.)

The effects of oxidation are like a domino effect that starts a whole cascade of events that ultimately wind up causing the body to be sick and age at a much faster rate. With this in mind, don't you think that it would be a good idea to control the rate of oxidation in your body?

If the skin cells oxidize over a period of time, the quality of the skin begins to change. People who have high levels of oxidation often deal with skin problems. Most people think of skin as just a covering or strictly a barrier that holds our contents inside. The truth is, the skin is the largest organ in the body. It is a highly sensitive and extremely complex organ that plays a dramatic role in the maintenance of our health and well-being. The skin is often a good indicator of what is really going on inside. When oxidative changes are prevalent in the inside of the body, those same effects can be also seen manifesting in the skin. Psoriasis, eczema, dry skin, rashes, spots, blemishes, premature aging, and skin cancers, can all be caused by oxidation affecting the internal structures also affecting the external. It is the degeneration of the skin and the collagen tissues in your body that make you age faster. How many times have you seen people who look perfectly normal go through a horrific event in their life? Perhaps they go through some traumatic ordeal, some crisis, or they undergo some kind of aggressive medical treatments, and you see them, maybe a month later, six months later, and they look like they have aged ten years. You can actually physically see the oxidative changes in their appearance. Just like you saw the apple and the shiny piece of metal degenerate right in front of your eyes! That is what excess oxidation can do to someone.

When the body starts breaking down and the physical structure starts to degenerate, nerve endings are stimulated. The nerve endings send electrical impulses to the brain just like an alarm system. When the brain is notified that the body parts are being damaged, it starts to respond. One of the first responses to initiate healing is the inflammatory response. Yes, good, old-fashioned swelling. When something is swollen or inflamed in the body, the next response is it produces pain. Pain is perceived in the brain, which, in turn, causes other compensatory responses in an attempt to protect the body from the further damage. In some cases, it might cause muscle spasms or stiffness and soreness. In other cases, it might cause joint pain and inflammation or aching and throbbing pain. If the injury is acute, it may cause intense debilitating pain with accompanying spasms and severe swelling and inflammation. When it comes to survival physiology, the body does not think or reason, it just reacts. Sometimes the reaction is not pleasant but may be necessary in order to preserve the damaged area.

> **One of the hardest things to convince someone of when they are suffering from the symptoms of pain is that it may be a necessary part of the healing process.**

Pain is nothing more than a reaction by the body in order to bring preservation to the part that is being affected. The unpleasant experience of pain most often drives us to do something to attempt to eliminate the pain. One of the hardest things to convince someone of when they are suffering from the symptoms of pain is that it may be a necessary part of the healing process. People are trained from a small child to think that pain is our enemy. There is constant instruction to "take this pill or drink that potion" whenever they experience any type of pain ranging anything from a stomachache, to back pain, to leg cramps, to a headache. Even though it is a hard concept to embrace, pain is our friend! It is what the body uses to notify us that there is a problem. Silencing pain is like putting ear plugs in when a fire alarm goes off. You may not have to deal with the irritating alarm but you will still have to deal with the damage caused by the fire. Covering up pain is not the answer.

The thing that needs to be accomplished is to try to control the oxidation and inflammation. The obvious question that needs to be answered is, "How do you do that?"

Well, God has thought of everything and since He knew that you would have to eat, breathe, and exercise, He also put things in nature's pharmacy called **antioxidants**. If you have the right amount and balance of antioxidants, you can eat, breathe, exercise, and age normally, and you do not have to worry about your body breaking down on you like the apple or the metal. Your body even has systems built in that are able to construct its own antioxidants as needed. Therefore, antioxidants are essential and crucial for longevity and vitality.

Oxidation levels can be monitored by using a **urinary oxidative stress test.** The sad truth is that if a large group of random people were selected and were tested, the highest percentage would test excessively high on the oxidative scale. Most people who get tested are usually shocked when they see how much oxidation they actually have in their bodies.

So what does all this mean? It means that when you have high levels of oxidation, when you try to exercise, or try to do a few physical chores around the house, and you push yourself a little extra, you get tired faster because your cells start breaking down. It means you have more pain after you exercise. You are more likely to have inflammation in your joints and soreness in your muscles, especially when you wake up in the morning. It may seem like something is always hurting, something is constantly wrong, or there is pain somewhere in the body all of the time. People find themselves making statements like, "It seems like I always get headaches," or "I stay exhausted," or even, "I don't know why this pain won't go away." These problems are commonly seen with people with high oxidation.

When oxidation levels are excessively high in the body, one of the first things that should be addressed is getting extra antioxidants into the system. For example, let us look at vitamin C (ascorbic acid). Vitamin C is a very powerful antioxidant. Let's say someone cuts up an apple into slices and puts them on a plate to serve at dinner later that evening. To prevent the apple from turning brown, they sprinkle it with ascorbic acid powder (vitamin C) because it is an "anti"-oxidant. What happens to the apple? It stays nice and fresh looking and is preserved because it is protected by the antioxidant effect of the vitamin C. That is what happens when we put vitamin C into our bodies. Just like the apple, our cells are preserved and protected by the antioxidant effect that keeps them safe and healthy. This same effect is produced every time we put any antioxidant into the body.

What do most metalworkers do to keep metal from oxidizing? They buy metal that is coated with zinc. Zinc is an antioxidant. If the metal is protected by the antioxidant rich zinc coating, the metal does not oxidize and stays protected from its damaging effects. If a little extra zinc is added to the diet, it protects our cells the same way. Adding antioxidant rich foods and supplementing with additional doses can protect the cells in the same way the apple and the metal were protected and preserved. They help to protect the cells from oxidizing. Fruits and vegetables are full of antioxidants and are the best way to consume them. The problem I often run into is the fact that a lot of people have food sensitivities, and eating certain fruits and vegetables may cause them more harm than good. If people have sensitivities to certain foods, even so-called healthy foods, those foods can cause oxidation and inflammation if consumed. That is why when some people try to clean up their diet and eat healthy, in some cases it makes them worse. Most of the people I have treated that have high levels of oxidation also have a fair amount of gut issues, food sensitivities being one that is prevalent.

Ingesting antioxidants into the body is a great first step in combating oxidation, but is only a small part of the solution for people with high oxidation levels. God equipped our bodies with antioxidant systems that actually manufacture antioxidants in the body's pharmacy. When these systems are working efficiently, the body is able to neutralize the excess oxidation keeping the body safe from its harmful effects. When someone is suffering from pain due to the effects of excessive oxidation, these systems should be one of the first things evaluated to make sure they are functioning properly. These antioxidant systems also serve a lot of other functions in the body as well, and need to be optimized at all costs.

Cholesterol, Lipoproteins, and Particle Size

Total cholesterol levels are a very ineffective way to diagnose the potential for cardiovascular disease. The most specific way to monitor whether cholesterol molecules are contributing to heart disease is to order a **VAP cholesterol blood test**. The VAP test assesses levels of all the blood lipids measured in a standard lipid profile (total **cholesterol**, LDL, HDL, VLDLs, and triglycerides), plus subclasses of lipids that are known or emerging risk factors for cardiovascular disease, such as LDL particle size and lipoprotein(a). Different types of cholesterol molecules are affected differently. The traditional thought used to be **high density lipids (HDLs)** were good and **low density lipids (LDLs)** were bad. The truth is, some HDLs are good and some HDLs are bad. The same goes for LDLs, some are good and some are bad. The designation of good and bad is determined by particle size and whether they are being oxidized or not. Some of the particles have serious consequences associated with their accumulation in the system. Particles like **VLDL3's** for example. Most people and even some doctors may have never heard of these and if they have, can probably not accurately describe their role in the body. The problem is that when these particles are present in high amounts in the system, they cause blood clots and put people at high risk for strokes. Does anyone want any extra blood clots floating around? The answer is obviously no. However, when you only get the routine cholesterol blood test results, the VLDL3's are not checked.

You would be surprised at the amount of blood tests I and my colleagues order that return with elevated levels of VLDL3's. This means there are people who are walking around that could be like potential time bombs waiting to go off, who are on the verge of having a stroke, and they have been told, "Oh, you are fine because your total cholesterol is normal." They may even feel more secure by knowing that their HDL's and LDLs look good as well. The problem with this scenario is nobody is looking deeper into their levels. A little bit of information can be good but too little can be disastrous. Knowing how to investigate thoroughly to find out what really causes diseases and disorders is what needs to happen if you want to prevent them. Let's look at another common problem and assess how we approach the solution.

> **A little bit of information can be good but too little can be disastrous.**

Most people have heard of the **formation of plaque**. When plaque builds up in the blood vessels it **can cause them to narrow, restrict, or even block the blood flow**. The blockage can cause a heart attack depriving the heart of vital oxygen. No one wants plaque to form in his or her arteries. The traditional way to prevent this from occurring is to take **statin drugs**. The only problem with this approach is these drugs don't stop the formation of plaque. When plaque samples were broken down and analyzed, the primary components found were LDL's, lipoprotein(a), IDL's and VLDL's. Statin drugs have very little, to perhaps no affect, on any of these components with the exception of total LDL (remember, some LDL fractions are beneficial). In a recent interview Professor Sherif Sultan, president of the International Society for Vascular Surgery, stated, "People are taking this drug to prevent a problem and are creating a disaster."

He also said, "Millions of people should stop taking the heart drugs because side effects outweigh possible benefits."

That's probably why there are some statistics that also show there are about as many people who have heart attacks and even worse problems while taking statin drugs than there are people not taking them at all. So my question is, why are people taking them? Statin drugs are known to produce severe muscle pain in the back and extremities as their side effects. If you are taking statin drugs and are experiencing pain, there's a high probability the medication is the cause of that pain. This is especially true if you didn't have any pain prior to taking them. There are many other safe alternatives to taking statin drugs that do not have these side effects associated with them. This will be covered in depth as you continue to read in the coming chapters. There are countless people who are suffering with debilitating pain that have no idea it is being caused by their medications. I am a firm believer in consulting a pharmacist or at least researching the side effects of any medication prior to taking it.

Why does everyone keep talking about total cholesterol? The statin drugs lower total cholesterol levels but lipoprotein(a) and the other components just discussed are unaffected. Elevated levels of certain ones of the small oxidized particles of LDLs quadruple someone's chances of having a heart attack. This is certainly an unwanted risk. However, if someone has high levels of lipoprotein(a), they are ten times more likely to have a heart attack. So why isn't everyone talking about that instead of total cholesterol? Lipoprotein(a) is almost never talked about. Have you ever heard of it? I bet I can tell you why you haven't. Statin drugs are ineffective in lowering lipoprotein(a); therefore the pharmaceutical companies don't spend the money to educate the public on the subject. What the public needs to be educated about is that research clearly shows that the correct levels of **niacin** added to the diet can normalize the levels of lipoprotein(a).[1]

Niacin also doesn't produce the painful side effects that the statins do. If you ever take niacin you should expect to get a niacin flush. Your face and ears might turn slightly red and feel a mild tingling in the face and extremities but this is normal and completely harmless. If you find that you are flushing too much, take one to two thousand milligrams of vitamin C with the niacin and it should minimize that flushing. Once the body gets used to taking it, the flushing should stop.

These are simple basic nutrients and are extremely effective. So why doesn't everyone get this information? The answer is quite simple: There is no patent on them.

Statin Drugs Can Cause Pain

When people take a statin drug it creates a deficiency of **Coenzyme Q10.** CoQ10 is a vital nutrient required by the body to produce and maintain energy. The drug blocks the CoQ10 cycle that facilitates the transfer of electrons to efficiently produce energy in the mitochondria of the cells, especially in your heart muscle, that makes it strong and healthy. Mitochondria are the little energy factories in the cell that create energy in order to do things like make your heart pump and your muscles to work efficiently. If someone has an elevated cholesterol level the most popular treatment of choice, is hands down, statin drugs. These drugs are proven to block the production of CoQ10. CoQ10 is found in practically every cell of your body. If statin drugs block this vital cycle, is it helping prevent disease or perhaps adding more risk factors? If you are currently taking a statin drug or have taken one in the past and are experiencing unexplained pain, you may want to consider taking some CoQ10 to prevent a potential deficiency and replenish the system to eliminate that pain. These medications can cause all kinds of pain syndromes. When my father was still alive he called me and said that his cardiologist put him on a statin drug. He asked my opinion and I explained to him about the risks and potential side effects in a very matter-of-fact manner. About a month later he called me and told me he was having trouble getting up to the house from the barn because he was having so much pain and weakness in his low back and legs. My father was very healthy and was quite strong and agile for his age. My mind immediately went back to the conversation we had a month prior. I asked him, "Have you been taking that statin drug?" After a long pause he replied, "Yes, I have." My reply was direct and straight to the point. "So how's that working out for you?" He immediately elected to come off of the medication and I recommended he take a combination of ubiquinol and ubiquinone (converted and unconverted forms of CoQ10) along with some neutraceuticals and nutrients to assist with reducing his systemic oxidation and inflammation. Within two weeks the pain was gone and he was fully recovered. He never had any other issues and actually a couple of weeks before he passed, he had a full blood workup and his levels were all normal.

Free Radicals

One of the most commonly overlooked causes of pain and inflammation is caused from a process called free radical pathology. **Free radicals** are unstable atoms that cause degenerative processes in the body from **reactive oxygen species (ROS)**. ROS is a hyper oxidation of processes in the body that lead to rapid cell damage. Free radicals are caused from the formation of these reactive oxygen species. This is just another process that leads to severe oxidation in the body.

When someone eats foods that are highly overcooked and over-processed, they are packed full of free radicals, especially oils. At fast food restaurants the oil cooks at high temperatures for hours, the fat molecules denature and make trans fats. These fats cause the formation of free radicals when consumed and cause damage to the cells. This process of oxidation produces inflammation and can lead to a cascade of damage all the way through the system. This can eventually lead to pain and soreness in muscles, joints, and collagen tissues.

People are walking around every day saying, "My neck hurts. My back hurts. My arms hurt. My shoulders hurt." Everything hurts. Why does it hurt? Free radicals damage all tissues. They damage blood vessels, organs, glands, the brain, very vital structures, and yes, they also damage joints and muscles. Joints and muscles are full of nerve endings and when they become damaged in any way, they are quick to report it to the brain. Pain and soreness are soon to follow. The other structures can be damaged but usually don't cause pain syndromes until they are damaged to the point of where their function is compromised. Therefore, many times muscle and joint pain caused from free radical damage can be an early sign to warn us that our entire body is being damaged.

What causes free radicals and how do we avoid them? Here's a list of five common sources from which free radicals are produced that most people don't realize cause free radical damage. There are all kinds of potential sources but these are a few of the main sources that lead to this highly destructive process.

1.The number one is smoking, both first or second-hand smoke. This one you probably saw coming, but the rest of them may catch you by surprise.

2. Health Supplements - Most people like to be thrifty and save money when shopping for products. When it's time to purchase health supplements, this is no exception to the rule. People who

are health savvy know that fish oils help to prevent oxidation in the body. However, guess where most people purchase them? They buy them in bulk at a cheap price, either online or in some of the major chain stores. This is a good example of, "you get what you pay for." Fish oils and EPA oils that you get in a large quantity very cheap are usually extremely high in **lipid peroxidase** (substances that cause excessive oxidation) because of the way they have been manufactured. Most of those oils are oxidized, and when someone consumes them they cause far more free radical damage than they could ever have potential to reduce. They are probably damaging you faster than they are repairing. Don't ever assume that nutrients at a bargain price are a better deal. Usually you get what you pay for. You should make sure that whatever you put in the body does what it's supposed to do instead of actually making the problem your taking it for worse.

3. Toxic chemicals are another source that causes free radical damage. From blue air on the horizon to tap water, our environment is full of chemicals. There is a large amount of preservatives in our foods. There are chemicals involved with so many things we do. People spray insect repellents and they don't bother to cover their nose and mouth. They use pesticides to kill the bugs in their gardens and don't wear gloves. They spray weeds with chemicals like glyphosphate (sold as Roundup by Monsanto) and get it on their skin, not realizing it is going right through into their systems where it causes damage to the exposed tissues. These toxic chemicals also damage the DNA of cells and can cause them to produce things like cancer, neurological disorders, or other serious diseases and disorders. It's quite common, when the cells' DNA is damaged this way, it may express a gene called an oncogene. This means that normal cells start to express as cancer. These genetic mutations can occur when there is physical damage that's done to the DNA. This is quite

common in exposure to intense stress, radiation, or extreme toxicity. If you have ever seen the spirals of DNA, they look like twisted ladders. When damage occurs within the DNA, it is like taking one of the ladders and splitting it down the middle of the rungs. When the DNA repairs itself it reconnects the rungs back together so it can heal. If as it comes back together it reconnects in the right pairing or coupling, then the structure is normal and the DNA will continue to express the same way it did before it was injured. However, if something injures it to the point where the rungs don't pair together the way they were previously, then the DNA will express itself differently than it should. DNA is what gives the instruction to the cells on how to produce new cells. If there is damaged DNA, it produces abnormal cells, or damaged cells, or defective cells or a system can no longer do what it needs to do at the rate it was doing it before.

Chemicals enter the body so fast sometimes that the person may not even realize that they were exposed. One example would be the moment you smell any harmful chemical. Simultaneously occurring at about the same time as you smell it, it's absorbed through the lungs and into your bloodstream. Once it is in the bloodstream, it is exposed to most all of the cells in your system. This means the system is exposed to the toxic effects causing cells, as well as DNA, to be damaged. Toxic chemicals are high free radical producers. This should make you think twice before spraying chemicals without a proper mask or using them without wearing gloves. The best approach is to avoid them altogether.

4. Electromagnetic frequencies (EMF) - There are all kinds of **electromagnetic frequency waves** bombarding you continually each and every day. We live in an electronic age. Cell phones, Bluetooth and WiFi-compatible devices are as common to wear as the clothes we put on each day. There are different types of radio, cell tower, cable, and electrical signals that are flying around us and through us

on a daily basis. The problem is, we really don't know what the long-term effects of this excessive electromagnetic frequency exposure (EMF) will be. Researchers are already reporting health issues of all kinds believed to be caused by it. Brain cancer and tumors are some of the most highly suspected currently. The National Toxicology Program (NTP), headquartered at NIEHS, just completed the largest animal study, to date, on cell phone radio frequency exposure.[2]

The study concluded that EMF from cell phones (and other 2G and 3G) devices were directly correlated with producing cancerous tumors in the heart, brain, and the adrenal glands of mice.

Oxidative stress occurs if the antioxidant defense system is unable to prevent the harmful effects of free radicals. Several studies have reported that exposure to EMF results in oxidative stress in many tissues of the body. Exposure to EMF is known to increase free radical concentrations in the body.[3] People don't seem to mind living with these devices constantly attached to their bodies. Common sense should tell us this can't be a good thing, but now science is proving it. The problem is the fact that we are so used to doing it, the assumption is if everyone is doing it then it must be okay. Nothing could be further from the truth. People used to think smoking was okay. Lots of people thought asbestos was okay. Many of those people died from cancer because they believed in the status quo. Doing what everyone else is doing is certainly not a practical nor safe way to prevent health problems. This type of exposure is now being shown to produce symptoms like fatigue, muscle soreness, depression, anxiety, restlessness, and even pain. I truly believe as time goes on researchers will continue to bring the proof that most of us already suspect about EMF to the forefront, so more strategies to prevent the damage can be developed. There are some practical ways to minimize this exposure.

A. Don't carry devices next to your body when you are not using them.

B. Turn off your devices when not using them.

C. Wear a multipolar magnet to neutralize the body's field.

D. Use a pulsed electromagnetic device to help balance the autonomic system.

E. Walk around barefoot at times allowing the feet to make direct contact with the earth, like walks on the beach or across the yard.

F. Take drives to places where there is no cell phone coverage and spend some time there.

G. Do an electromagnetic detox where you fast the use of all of your devices for a few hours each day.

H. Do not sleep with your cell phone or other devices.

These are a few steps to get you moving in the right direction. Come up with some ideas of your own and implement them as well.

5. Advanced Glycation End-products (AGE) - Modern diets are largely heat-processed and as a result contain high levels of **advanced glycation end products (AGEs)**. These end products are known to contribute to increased oxidant stress and inflammation, which are linked to the recent epidemics of diabetes and cardiovascular disease.[4] They are most commonly found in fatty meats, especially those cooked over high heat (which produces potential carcinogens such as heterocyclic amines, or HCAs) and in fried or highly processed foods such as chips and French fries. AGEs block nitric oxide activity in the endothelium and cause the production of reactive oxygen species.[5] Glycation and oxidative stress are closely

linked, and are often referred to as "glycoxidation" processes. All glycation steps generate oxygen-free radicals, some of these steps being common with these of lipid peroxidation. AGEs bind to membrane receptors such as RAGE, and induce an oxidative stress and a pro-inflammatory status.[6] What does all of this science mean? It means when you consume these products, they cause a bombardment of free radicals to be released causing oxidative damage and inflammation throughout the entire body. For the average person this usually winds up producing pain and discomfort some place in the body. AGEs accumulate in an age-related fashion in the brain and other organs of the central nervous system of individuals in many different neurodegenerative diseases, including Alzheimer, Parkinson, and other less common diseases.[7]

The best way to prevent AGEs from building up in the system is to avoid the foods that contain them. Increasing the antioxidant systems and consumption of antioxidants also reduces them. They damage cells and cause you to age prematurely. Yes, AGEs age you! This will give you something to think about before you reach for that next bag of chips.

System Transport

Have you ever wondered how things move around in the body? The nutrients, oxygen, and all of the components that are required by the body to stay alive are all packed inside of the blood. The Bible says that the life is in the blood. Have you ever wondered what blood is? What does blood do? What is it for? Why do we have blood vessels? The answer is quite obvious., The cells need to exchange vital substances, from hormones and nourishment to waste removal. The body needs to move substances to and from the cells. The blood system is like a system of little transport tracks; so the blood is nothing more than a physical transport mechanism to carry things to cells all over the body. That is how the cells are able to replenish and make new ones. The blood is crucial for survival, so functions like circulation are equally as important. Since the heart is the pump that pushes the life system around its function must be optimized in order to keep up with the demand. How about the vessels that carry the precious life that is in the blood? It's important that those vessels are clear, free-flowing, and smooth so everything that needs to be delivered can travel in and out of the cells without impedance. In the **body**, the amino acid arginine changes into **nitric oxide**. **Nitric oxide** is a powerful neurotransmitter that helps blood vessels relax and also improves circulation. Some evidence shows that arginine may help improve blood flow in the arteries of the heart.

Circulation starts with arteries and connects to even smaller vessels called arterioles, which connect to capillary beds. The vessels are like major highways going down to streets; from the streets, into the capillary beds, which are like loading docks; and they load things out to the cells, they take things back and have exchange in millions of capillary beds around your entire system; and that exchange is going on all day. That is what makes you be able to function. That is what makes you healthy, or in some cases, not healthy.

If your loading docks are blocked, do you suppose there is much exchange going on? When there is no exchange, it means there is probably not too much happening in the cell; so then the cell starts to die. If vessels are not moving blood at the rate they should, or if the blood is not traveling down at the speed, quality, or volume it should, parts of the body become deprived. If this process is continued for an extended period of time, what do you suppose happens to the cells in those areas? Perhaps they might die? More disease? More disorders? The answer seems pretty obvious.

So with this in mind, the last thing we want to happen is for our circulation to become impeded or impaired. Poor circulation can cause anything from sore muscles and cramps to full-blown pain and inflammation. Blood flow can be determined by a number of factors. Poorly digested or undigested food molecules (especially proteins), altered clotting factors, blood vessel compression or occlusion, atherosclerosis or arteriosclerosis, tight restricted muscles, and excessive buildup of toxins, are just a few things that can cause restrictive blood flow. Due to scientific discoveries of various natural enzymes, some of these problems can be resolved and in some cases possibly reversed.

Enzymes from Nature's Pharmacy

Serrapeptase is an unusual enzyme that comes from the serratia, a bioactive bacteria that lives inside the gut of silkworms. These serratia produce serrapeptase, an enzyme known to dissolve proteins. The serrapeptase dissolves the silk cocoon, allowing the silkworms to evacuate when it's time. What's really amazing is the fact that it has been used successfully in humans to reduce inflammation, decrease pain and soreness, and also to help to dissolve scar tissue. Serrapeptases benefits come from its ability to dissolve protein and fibrin substances. When taken at the correct dosage it can actually help someone to heal faster. Dr. Hans Napier did extensive work in the study of this amazing enzyme. He mentions that the first reliable results come from taking serrapeptase for 6-8 months. He also stated that some of his patients taking it for up to 18 months were still displaying results.[8] The acceptable effective dosage is between 30,000-40,000 spu/eu per day on a completely empty stomach. One of its most remarkable functions is that it affects only non-living tissue such as the proteins in the silk cocoon. According to Dr. Napier, in the human body, serrapeptase dissolves only dead tissues such as the old fibrous layers that clog the linings of our arteries and dangerously restrict the flow of blood and oxygen to the brain. It is also extremely useful in keeping arterial deposits from building up again after angioplasty or coronary bypass surgery has been performed. He also stated that many of his patients have shown improved blood flow through their previously constricted arteries confirmed by ultrasound examination.

Nattokinase is an enzyme that is extracted from a popular Japanese food called natto. The process consists of adding beneficial bacteria, *Bacillus Natto*, to boiled soybeans until they become fermented. Dr. Hiroyuki Sumi discovered the enzyme in 1980. His research compiled with additional research, including seventeen published studies in Japan and in the U.S., show that nattokinase supports the normal blood clotting mechanism, supports healthy blood viscosity, and helps maintain healthy blood flow. It's a powerful enzyme that breaks down the fibrin that causes clots as well as enhances the body's natural production of plasmin (enzyme that also dissolves fibrin clots). Web M.D. states on their website that nattokinase "thins the blood" and helps break up clots. The typical recommended effective dose is 2000 FU (fibrin units) of nattokinase a day. If you are on a blood thinner or have a bleeding disorder you should always consult your physician before taking this or any other blood-thinning agent.

Lumbrokinase is a typically well-tolerated and very safe fibrin dissolving enzyme that comes from earthworms. In 1991 Dr. Mihara and other scientists in Japan successfully extracted and characterized a group fibrinolytic enzymes from the earthworm species, Lumbricus rubellus. These enzymes are capable of degrading both plasminogen-rich and plasminogen-free fibrin (clot-forming substances). These enzymes were collectively named Lumbrokinase (LK) after the genus name for earthworm, Lumbricus. LK is very specific to fibrin and does not cause excessive bleeding. LK has shown therapeutic use in dissolving clots, lowering whole blood viscosity, and reducing platelet aggregation (clumping of clot-forming cells), all of which promote improved blood circulation. Currently they are widely used clinically in China as a thrombolytic agent to dissolve clots. It has also been used successfully for breaking down biofilms (thick clumps of gut bacteria) associated with Lyme disease patients. It's especially effective for improving circulation in the small capillary beds throughout the body and extremities. This can improve the flow and distribution of nutrients to the cells.

Gut Health

The digestive system is referred to as the **gastrointestinal system** which includes all of the digestive and elimination organs, glands, and digestive tract from the mouth all the way to the anus. The digestive tract is properly called the **alimentary tract** and is also commonly referred to as the "**gut**." It is an area where inflammation can originate and can be a source of perpetual inflammation in a lot of people. I believe it is a root source of many, and I said *many*, diseases and disorders that people would not typically associate them with. In order to embrace that statement there needs to be an enlightening discussion about the gut.

The easiest way to explain it is to visualize it as a tube. It is a tubular structure. This tube has linings all the way from the mouth down to the anus made up of tissue called endothelium.

How do we make this body that we live in healthy? How do we keep it alive? How does it get the fuel that it needs to function? Very simply: from *food*. There is something important to know about food: food is a wonderful thing because it becomes fuel, fuel becomes energy, and energy sustains life. However, if the food isn't broken down and utilized properly, it can cause more harm than good.

Let us take a little journey through the digestive system in order to better understand how our bodies turn food into fuel. Food is consumed as the mouth takes a bite of it. Immediately a digestive enzyme called **salivary amylase** is released into the mouth through the saliva. This enzyme begins breaking down carbohydrates on contact. The powerful jaws use the muscles of mastication to chew the food, and large particles of the food are broken into smaller particles. This has to take place because the large particles are too big to go into the cell to be used as fuel. Next, the swallowing process initiates and uses the muscles in the throat to push particles down through the **esophagus**, all the way to the **stomach**. When it gets to the stomach there is **hydrochloric acid (HCL)** waiting there to start digesting the stuff that has been chewed to break it down into even smaller particles. When the particles get smaller there is more surface area revealed which makes it easier for the acid to break them down and the process continues. There are also other digestive enzymes in the gastric juice like **pepsin**, **rennin**, and **mucous** to further break the food down until it finally goes to the next chamber which is called the **duodenum**.

This is where the **pancreas** gets involved. Most people know that the head of the pancreas produces **insulin** to facilitate sugar. What they usually do not know is that the tail of the pancreas produces **digestive enzymes** that digest proteins, carbohydrates, and fats (called **pancreatic enzymes**). When the food travels into the duodenum these pancreatic enzymes are released into the same chamber and start to digest the remaining particles so they can be absorbed into the cells and turn it into energy. If the pancreas becomes fatigued or dysfunctional, it does not produce adequate amounts of enzymes. If there are not enough enzymes then the food cannot be completely digested. This obviously can cause deficiencies, but there are also other problems that can also occur as a result. Incomplete digestion can cause food sensitivities that produce inflammatory bowel syndromes leading to a variety of pain syndromes. It can also cause powerful inflammatory chemicals called **leukotrienes** to be released into the system causing inflammation and pain throughout the body. Complete digestion is extremely important in the reduction of pain and inflammation, especially those who suffer from chronic pain. The use of pancreatic enzymes can be extremely effective for eliminating these types of pain syndromes by correcting the problem that causes the process.

When people have high sugar diets, they often complain of reflux, **G.E.R.D.** Individuals who have G.E.R.D. keep burping up acid. Those who have acid reflux and have been dealing with it on a daily basis can stop this process by simply taking the refined carbohydrates out of the diet. Instead of depending on antacids and proton pump inhibitors that ultimately make the problem worse, why not just fix the problem? Stop consuming sugar products and stay away from refined foods. Stop eating and drinking the things that convert immediately to carbohydrates, and the reflux should stop. The symptoms should stop within three to five days and the reflux should be gone. No more sleeping on wedged pillows, no more getting expensive prescriptions because the over-the-counters no longer work, no longer should you have to live on antacids.

Calcium is a very useful nutrient. What do you suppose calcium has to have in order to break it down so the body can absorb it? It has to have hydrochloric acid (HCL). If someone takes antacids or proton pump inhibitors it neutralizes the stomach acid (HCL). Without HCL, calcium cannot be digested. Calcium can be consumed in high quantities but it cannot do anything for the system if it is not broken down. When someone's system becomes deficient in calcium, they can experience symptoms like cramping, muscle spasms, muscle weakness, irritability, pins and needles sensations, as well as bone, joint, and, muscle pain. Osteoporosis, neurological consequences, and musculoskeletal complaints can also ensue. The world is practically living on antacids. Another problem we face as humans is that as we age, especially as we enter our fifties and sixties, our bodies do not produce the same amount of hydrochloric acid that it once did. That is why acid indigestion among the elderly is so common. As someone ages his or her diet starts to change. They start eating softer and softer foods, by nature and by recourse, because that is the natural progression of how things happen. When the elderly population takes an antacid, they are really setting themselves up for trouble. Who do you suppose has the highest occurrence of osteoporosis? Yes, the elderly.

Often when people have chronic acid problems like G.E.R.D., heartburn, or acid indigestion, I recommend they take HCL. That's right, not an antacid but instead I give them acid, betaine hydrochloride. When they take it with their meals, the problem usually goes away rather quickly, because the body no longer has to overcompensate. Instead of hindering the digestive process we have enhanced it. When stomach acid levels are normalized, calcium can be properly digested and utilized by the body. Therefore, the symptoms, including reflux, spasms, cramps, and pain, subside as a result.

The key to digesting food is the acid needs to be intact to break it down and there has to be enough pancreatic enzymes to complete digestion. If someone has excessive flatulence (gas out of the bottom, not belching), that means that they probably have a digestive enzyme problem and taking pancreatic enzymes should stop it. If someone has gas from the top like belching and burping, then it is usually a hydrochloric acid problem. A little betaine hydrochloride usually takes care of that. Getting off the refined carbohydrates, eating raw foods full of enzymes also makes a huge difference.

Proteins

In my first book, *Healing by Design*, I explained how our society has turned into a group of carboholics, consuming too many of the wrong types of carbohydrates that cause all kinds of health consequences including becoming addicted to the very foods that cause the problem. This carboholic lifestyle has left many people's bodies in a very unhealthy state. Chronic pain syndromes can be one of the by-products of this lifestyle. For the purpose of this discussion, let us delve a little deeper into what else happens to cause these pain syndromes so those who are suffering from it can STOP THE PAIN.

The body has to have **amino acids** in order to heal its tissues and structures. Without them nothing can regenerate and therefore the body cannot repair itself. Remember, when the rate of damage exceeds the rate of repair, the end product is degeneration, inflammation, and finally disease. One of the first symptoms to show up when this starts to take place is pain. The digestive system breaks down proteins into amino acids so the body can repair itself. If the proteins are not properly digested then the amino acids are not available and the repair process is inhibited. Protein digestion is essential in the treatment of pain-related illness. When people have problems digesting proteins or have chronic pain syndromes, I often recommend they supplement with amino acids along with treating the digestive issue. Those who athletically train, work out with weights, play sports, or even have jobs that require excessive lifting or straining, should all consider adding amino acid supplementation to their diets. People who stay sore most of the time should as well. Twenty to thirty grams daily of amino acid supplementation is not uncommon, all the way up to forty to fifty grams depending upon the intensity of the activity. Patients report to me on a regular basis how many of their aches, pains, and soreness improve after they add amino to their diets. Another really effective addition for people who suffer with pain, especially chronic pain, is supplementing with **collagen protein**. It's one of my absolute favorites. The tissues that support the body, including the ones in the skin that get wrinkled, are made up of collagen. My own experience, both personally and professionally, is that consuming collagen protein is almost like drinking from the fountain of youth. I take it nearly every day. I am still able to train at the gym at a very intense level and also play head to head tennis with my son who has a scholarship and plays as the number one seed on his college team. Taking collagen protein enables me to recover from this type of intense activity without experiencing any pain in my body. If I get busy with my schedule and forget to take it regularly, Mother Nature is quickly there to remind me that I am not as young as I used to be. However, if I am consistent in taking it, I continue to enjoy my youthful ability. Consuming thirty to forty grams can prove to be highly effective in many cases. It may be a good idea to add pancreatic enzymes at the same time to help ensure the proteins get broken down into amino acids that the body desperately needs for repair. People who suffer with joint pain and/or stiffness and soreness usually greatly benefit from this combination. Adding joint compound, Mega EPAs, and Infla-ox makes it even more effective.

Fats

The great lie that most people have been taught is that fats are bad. The reason for this belief is that when people think about fat, they think about the kind that shows up around the waistline. That kind of fat is stored fat with a bunch of little estrogen factories in it. That kind shows up when the wrong kind of foods or the wrong balance of foods are introduced into the diet. Eating fat doesn't make someone fat any more than eating steak makes someone a cow. Fats are a very important part of the diet. When people have insatiable appetites, cravings, and a lack of energy, these are all signs of a lack of eating the right quantity of good fats. One of the first complaints people have when they go on diets to lose weight is that they are hungry. There's nothing worse than having to starve to lose weight. When someone adds the right amount of good quality fats to their diet the hunger stops. Fat calories produce two-and-one-quarter times the amount of energy than other sources do, so it stands to reason that they can be very beneficial for people who have had long-term problems where higher energy levels are required to overcome those problems. From slow metabolisms to chronic pain syndromes, the correct amount of quality fats can sometimes be the game changer when added to the diet. The obvious question that should come to mind is, "What are the right kind of fats to eat?" There are many choices, but I am going to list a few that research and clinical experience has proven to me make a difference.

> **Eating fat doesn't make someone fat any more than eating steak makes someone a cow.**

Good Sources of Fat:

1. **Flax seed** and **flax seed oil**

2. **Avocado** and **avocado oil**

3. **Cold water fish** and **fish oil**

4. **Coconut** and **coconut oil**

5. **Olives** and **olive oil**

6. **Chia seed** and **chia seed oil**

When the linings of cells and joints are deprived of the proper fats they begin to degenerate and become inflamed. This harmful process takes place not only because the right kind of fats aren't present to repair them, but also because there are too many of the wrong kind that damages them. What if you sent a construction crew into your house to repair it and they did more damage than they did to repair? Wouldn't that make things worse? It's bad enough the first problem didn't get fixed, but worse yet, the crew that was supposed to help the problem just added to it. That is what it is like every time you consume bad fats. The repairing process gets hindered and the linings break down faster than they can be repaired. Swapping good fats for the bad ones is a must in getting rid of chronic inflammatory processes in the body.

Digesting Fats

Consuming the right fats is crucial for good health but even more important is the ability to digest and assimilate them properly. Here's a quick synopsis on how the body digests fats. The **liver** makes a substance called **bile**. It stores it in the **gallbladder**, which concentrates it about twenty to thirty times, making it much stronger, and releases it right into the **duodenum** where it mixes with the **pancreatic enzymes**. The bile and the bile salts break down the fats so the digestion process is complete.

If you do not have a good bile system or if the gallbladder is full of sludge or full of stones, and it is not functioning properly, the fats do not get broken down properly. This can cause people to feel tired after they eat, especially after eating a fatty meal. Fatty stools, diarrhea, stomach and bowel pain, and even mid back pain and right sided parascapular pain can all manifest from poor fat digestion due to this condition.

Fats need to be digested properly in order to provide lubrication in the body. If they are not breaking down, the joints may not get the proper amount of lubrication they need to stay healthy. Without proper lubrication the joints dry out and can become painful, stiff, and will most likely develop some form of arthritis if the problem is not corrected. Other parts of the body may suffer as well causing things like dry, brittle hair, dry skin, and brittle nails.

There may be plenty of fats in the diet, but if you are not breaking them down properly the body cannot use them to heal the way they are designed to. I am an avid supporter of eating the healthier fats but if they are not getting digested properly, the problems and the pain continue. There are so many occasions when patients told me that they had been eating healthy diets and were including good fats, oils, and essential fatty acids, but their symptoms and pain did not improve or maybe even got worse. How can this be?

When foods are not properly digested they can become a burden on the body even when they are healthy choices. That is why it is so important to have optimal bile and gallbladder function to assist us in breaking down fats completely. Doing something as simple as a **gallbladder flush** to cleanse out the sludge along with a simple herbal and nutraceutical cleanse for the liver can have a profound effect on our health.

The gallbladder flush is simple to do.

[See Figure 1 on Next Page]

Figure 1

GALLBLADDER FLUSH		
DAY 1 - Regimen	**DAY 2 - Regimen**	**DAY 3 - Regimen**
No Food Drink 1 Gallon Apple Juice **Smaller 8 to 12oz portions during the day** **Drink water to hydrate if needed.**	No Food Drink 1 Gallon Apple Juice **Smaller 8 to 12oz portions during the day** **Drink water to hydrate if needed.**	Gallbladder will release its contents and flush occurs in the morning.
DAY 1 - EVENING	**DAY 2 - EVENING**	
Normal Bedtime Routine	Modified Bedtime Routine **Mix and drink before bedtime 1/2 cup of extra fine virgin olive oil, (it has to be the first pressing) and 1/2 cup of Lemon Juice (fresh squeezed)** Sleep on Your Right Side	

Drink one gallon of apple juice (preferably fresh squeezed or apple cider) per day for two days. Divide it up into eight to twelve ounce glasses and spread it out throughout the day. Do not eat any food during this time, just the apple juice. Water is allowed if more hydration is needed. At the end of the second day, when it is time to go to bed, take a half a cup of extra fine virgin olive oil, (it has to be the first pressing) and a half cup of lemon juice (preferably fresh squeezed) and mix them together. Drink it down, go to bed, and sleep on your right side. When you wake up in the morning, the gallbladder should release its contents and the flush will take place.

The sludge, and even small stones if present, should expel itself out of the gallbladder so the bile can return to its proper concentration.

It is a simple, inexpensive way to clean that system out. Following right behind the cleanse, doing an **organic coffee enema** can also be extremely beneficial to complete the process. Coffee enemas are an excellent way to promote good elimination and can also produce a powerful detox effect in the body.

Figure 2

ORGANIC COFFEE ENEMA

HYDRATE	SUPPLIES TO PURCHASE	2 DAYS AFTER
Hydration is important. Drink plenty of filtered water the day you will administer the enema.	Enema Kit Sieve to Strain Coffee Organic Coffee **Medium to large grind is preferred to avoid grounds in the enema.** **Grind and airtight refrigerate.** **DIRECTIONS** Boil Distilled//Filtered Water Add Desired Amount of Coffee **1-2 teaspoons to start.** **Strain coffee using sieve.** Add Cool Water to Mixture **Prepare 4 cups total.** **Verify mixture is lukewarm or below.** **Pour 2 cups into enema bag** Lie Down to Administer **Keep enema bag higher than body.** **Retain contents for 10-15 Minutes.** **Release on toilet.**	Flush toxins from the body. Drink plenty of filtered water a few days after you have administered the enema.

To get started make sure you purchase an enema kit which is easily obtained online. You'll also need a sieve for straining the coffee.

Next, grind some fresh organic whole bean coffee. A large to medium grind is typical. If you grind your coffee too finely, the grounds will pass through the sieve, and you'll have grounds in your enema. This is not a big concern, but a ground-free enema is preferred.

Grind all the coffee in a bag at once and store it in an air-tight container in the refrigerator to keep it fresh.

Bring the filtered or distilled water to a boil, add the desired amount of coffee, and simmer for 10 minutes. (1-2 teaspoons to start so you don't detox too quickly.)

Then strain the coffee through the sieve, add enough cool filtered or distilled water to equal 4 cups, and make sure your coffee + water mixture is at body temperature or below (lukewarm, not hot). Once it's at the right temperature, you're ready to do the enema. Start the enema by pouring half (2 cups) of your liquid into the enema bag administering it and retaining it for about 10-15 minutes. It's much easier to lie down while doing the enema keeping the bag higher than the body while administering the enema. After holding the contents for the allotted amount of time, you then sit on the toilet and release the remaining contents into the toilet bowl. The enema is complete. You can increase the amount of coffee in the enema once you establish toleration. It's not uncommon for people to use upward of 3-4 tablespoons to every 4 cups of coffee in those who have slowly worked themselves up through the detox process. If you do too much too fast you may develop some unpleasant symptoms such as nausea, vomiting, skin rash, or hives, etc. Start slow and work yourself up slowly so you don't have a negative reaction. Drink plenty of filtered water the day of and the following couple of days after doing the enema to help the body to flush the toxins through the system.

When the stomach acids are normalized, the pancreatic enzymes are plentiful, the bile and bile salts are at their proper concentrations. Then the food can be broken down completely so its nutrients can be absorbed as it travels through the small intestine. The only thing left over should be the waste products and all of the stuff that the body couldn't use.

Cholesterol

We need to talk about what happens when fats become oxidized. We eat a lot of fats in our diet. Let's face it, the American diet is full of fats, and if they start to oxidize, that is a recipe for disaster. When you oxidize fats, they start to congeal and to get hard. This is what makes cholesterol particles dangerous. In the vessels they cause damage to the linings that causes the formation of plaque. The inappropriate intake of dietary fats, excessive drinking of soft drinks, insulin resistance, and other poor lifestyle choices that produce excessive oxidative stress, lead to the accumulation of hepatic triglyceride accumulation in the liver. When the oxidized fats accumulate on the liver they cause a fatty liver. This condition is called non-alcoholic fatty acid liver disease (NAFLD). It resembles the same type of damage to the liver usually caused by excessive alcohol consumption. However, you don't have to be an alcoholic or even drink alcohol to have NAFLD.

It is a very destructive process when good healthy fats, as well as other fats, are being oxidized in the body and start to accumulate in places where they affect the body's function. Interestingly enough, **olive oil** consumption reverses the mechanisms that cause NAFLD by lowering NFkB activation, decreasing oxidation, and improving insulin resistance by reducing the level of inflammatory cytokines.[9] These mechanisms are fundamental in the cause and proliferation of many diseases and disorders in the body and will be explained in an easily understood format by the time you finish reading this book.

Have you ever had a physician review your blood work or a loved one's, and report to you that the cholesterol levels were elevated? Most of the time a statin drug is prescribed without any further evaluation. The problem is that cholesterol can elevate for a lot of reasons and some of the things that cause it can be potentially more harmful than the elevation itself. For example, one primary mechanism of cholesterol is as an antioxidant in the body, mainly HDL. With that in mind, if someone has elevated cholesterol levels, perhaps they have high levels of oxidation in their body and the cholesterol is elevating in an effort to lower the harmful oxidizing effect. In this scenario, is cholesterol really the bad guy? Most often elevated cholesterol gets blamed for heart disease when, truthfully, there are other underlying issues that need to be addressed. It is not the cholesterol that is causing the problem; it is the oxidation that is doing the damage. The cholesterol is trying to fix the problem, and people are taking drugs to try to lower the thing that is trying to help them. For example, if you see a fire you will also see a lot of firemen around that fire. If there was a test to evaluate the number of firemen at a fire and it came back as a higher than normal number, what would that tell you? You can blame the damage that is being caused on the firemen, or you can look deeper and see it is really the fire that needs to be dealt with. Cholesterol is like the firemen in this example and oxidation is the fire. It is the oxidation that needs to be dealt with and the higher number of firemen will reduce as the fire does.

Fats are categorized as high-density lipids (HDL's) and low-density lipids (LDL's). High-density lipids have a lot of protein and a little fat. We like the high density lipids because they are healing and the proteins in those lipid complexes break down into amino acids and deliver healing nutrients to the body. They are considered to be very good fats. The LDL's are most often considered to be the bad fats. Well, they are not really bad fats. They are good fats, but they can turn to bad fats. LDLs, or low-density lipids, mean they have a lot of fat and a little protein. The low-density lipids are the big fluffy fats and are like beach balls, and they move along through the vessels with a swabbing action, and actually help heal the intima linings inside of your blood vessels. These molecules are categorized by fractionation and are named based on their particle size.

The problem begins when they become oxidized. They get small and hard like billiard balls. Blood is pushed around the blood vessels at the speed of about a couple hundred miles an hour. What do you suppose happens when little small hard billiard balls (oxidized fats) start continually slamming into the sides of those vessels? Damage! When the body attempts to heal these damaged vessels, it forms plaque, which serves as a patch. Next comes the plaque build-up, which gets to the point where those small fat particles begin to work themselves through the intima lining and lodge between it and the muscle layer. Macrophages work like Pac-Man to devour these fats causing them to swell into what are called foam cells. These foam cells swell up causing the blood vessel to close off and narrow that vessel. This condition is called atherosclerosis. Which type of fats would you rather have in your vessels, beach balls or billiard balls? The billiard balls are the small particle sized fats; so cardiovascular disease is really more about particle size due to the oxidization of fats and really has nothing to do with total cholesterol levels.

That means one day you might be walking out to the mailbox thinking you are perfectly healthy, and all of a sudden you get a pain in your chest. The next thing you know you wind up in the ER and the doctors have to put in a stent. What are they doing? They are going into the blood vessel crammed full of billiard balls that the macrophages turned into foam cells causing compression of the vessel, and they are spreading it apart returning blood flow. It does save your life, but doesn't solve the long-term problem. The next step after the crisis is over should be to do what is necessary to get rid of the billiard balls. It is important to understand the cause of these conditions like this so you know what to do in case this ever happens to you, your family, or your friends. If you understand it, it shouldn't frighten you. You realize what the problem is and you understand how you got it. People who have this underlying condition many times get many warning signs such as neck, jaw, upper back and shoulder pain, chest pain, trouble catching their breath, numbness or tingling down the arms, to name a few of the symptoms. These often get ignored instead of going to the family physician and getting them checked out. There's a saying in our profession: "Don't let the patient die from the symptoms while you're treating the cause." If you are having any of these symptoms, please get them evaluated first. The next thing you need to learn is what you need to do to prevent it and possibly reverse it. Of course the best cure is always prevention.

> **Don't let the patient die from the symptoms while you're treating the cause.**

Heart disease is still the number one killer in America despite the efforts to prescribe medications to combat it. That is because mainstream healthcare has not been addressing the cause of the problem. The LDL cholesterol particles also serve as an antioxidant considered bad because they are shuttled to the blood vessel membrane to work along with vitamin C to serve as an antioxidant to heal the inflamed and oxidized damaged blood vessel linings. The

HDL cholesterol particles are considered good because they are shuttled away from the vessel membranes toward the liver in which case they don't accumulate in the vessels. No one wants plaque to build up in their arteries but LDLs are not the cause, they are just a sign for those who understand how this works, that there is a specific problem that needs corrected. Targeting the particles that are attempting to resolve the problem by lowering LDLs is not the answer. The answer is to target what's causing the damage (oxidation/inflammation) so there won't be a reason for them to be shuttled to the vessels in the first place. Oxidation and inflammation are the cause and they do not affect only the cardiovascular system. The entire body is affected by the destructive process, which spawns all types of disorders and conditions. These conditions damage cells, which, in turn, cause pain. The moral of the story is you need to prevent the fats from being oxidized in order to prevent them from being harmful to the system. So if we are taking our antioxidants, at least the fats are going to be significantly more resistant to oxidation.

When fats are ingested, they need to be broken down completely by the digestive system in order to prevent them from turning into harmful substances. When you burn a fat you burn a fat molecule, you get two-and-a-quarter times more energy than any other molecule in the body, so it would be better to use those for fuel. Right? Fats can be a very efficient source of energy. However, if you do not utilize them, they potentially can cause all kinds of problems in your body.

Gallbladder Function

The liver is your detoxification organ. It makes bile. Bile is golden brown. It is then put into the gallbladder, the gallbladder then concentrates it, and makes it much more potent and stronger changing it to green bile. It can then be released into the duodenum, which is an important part of your digestive tract where the digestion of fats can take place. The bile needs to be fully concentrated to get adequate breakdown of the fats, so you have to make sure that the liver and the gallbladder are working efficiently. It is quite common for people to get sludge in their gallbladders, and in many cases, gallstones are formed. This can cause fatty stools, symptoms after eating foods with high fat content, and even cause pain, especially sharp pain under or around the right shoulder blade.

There are herbal and nutritional detoxifications that you can do for the liver and gallbladder to help cleanse out this sludge, which can be a good option (dandelion, beet root, fenugreek, artichoke, etc.). The technique I have used for years in clinical practice is the Gallbladder Flush previously discussed. [See diagram p.100] This is an all-natural flush that has almost no cost involved, takes two days, and can provide some pretty impressive results. I have had many patients report to me that they have much more energy, their digestive issues go away, and many of their chronic pain issues disappear after doing this flush.

For right at thirty years, I have been recommending this cleanse to my patients and have never had anyone have a problem with doing the flush. Some people will say, "What if this happens or what if that happens?" The answer is, "I don't know. I have never had that happen." What I can offer is this: The patients I have recommended it to have done remarkably well. The choice is yours. You can choose not to do it and live with sludge in your gallbladder and potentially have digestive problems that can cause you health problems, or you can flush it out and, hopefully, have a good experience and potentially improve how you feel and function. There are also nutraceuticals that you can take that can help you break down fats more efficiently as well.

This book is designed to offer you some valid health strategies to help empower you to be able to **STOP THE PAIN** in your life. After you finish it from cover to cover you are going to realize that a lot of diseases come from your gut and digestive dysfunction.

Breaking down fats completely for digestion and assimilation is imperative for a normal functional metabolism and repair. The dispersement of these digested fats throughout the body are critical for healing and repair. Listed here is a collection of nutrients that the body uses to accomplish this task. These are only brief explanations to allow you to have a better understanding of how they all work together to enhance fat digestion.

Lecithin (phosphatidylcholine) is a fat emulsifier. What is an emulsifier? It is something that breaks down fat. Perhaps you have heard of Dawn dishwashing soap. If you put it in the dishwater, it breaks down the fat so it does not stick to the dishes. That is what an emulsifier does. Of course, you would not want to consume a dish soap so lecithin is a good choice to use in the digestive tract as an emulsifier of fats. It is able to work in your body, safely and effectively. That is how God made it. When you consume lecithin, it breaks fat down into nice, little, absorbable fat molecules. This allows the fats to be utilized by the cells instead of building up in the system.

Acetyl L- Carnitine (ALC) is extremely important for the digestion and assimilation of fats. It is the number one fat-burning amino acid in the body. It is an amino acid that turns fat into fuel. Isn't that what everyone wants to do, burn fat? The importance of ALC assisting in the assimilation and metabolism of fats is the same as having insulin assist in the assimilation and metabolism of sugars, ultimately driving them into the muscles for fuel. Anyone who has trouble metabolizing fats should want to include some additional ALC supplementation into their diet.

Conjugated Linoleic Acid (CLA) is a vitally important fatty acid that is found in beef. Some people, for whatever reason, do not like to have high beef diets. If you are one of those people, it is okay not to eat beef; but you still need that fatty acid, CLA. It is outstanding because it actually helps you burn fat; but it must come from the diet. Your body cannot manufacture it, so you have to get it from your diet or supplement if you are not going to eat red meats. There is an animal study that showed as little as point five percent (.5%) CLA added to the diet can reduce cancerous tumors by 50 percent. With that in mind, don't you think that it might be a good thing to add it into your diet? It also improves insulin resistance by increasing the effectiveness of alpha lipoid acid. What is insulin resistance? It is when you have eaten sugar for so long that the receptors now are resistant to it and you have to keep making more and more insulin, until pretty soon your pancreas wears out and you become a diabetic. Studies have shown that when you add CLA to the diet, it helps improve the function of alpha lipoic acid and helps to improve insulin resistance, which helps to desensitize those receptors so they do not require as much insulin. When working with physicians to help diabetics with their diets in an effort to lower or even get them completely off of their medications, the insulin resistance issue has to be addressed.

Essential Fatty acids are essential nutrients derived from dietary intake of fats. They are an important source of energy for the body, and serve a variety of other biologic functions. Greater dietary intake of **omega-3 polyunsaturated fatty acids (PUFAs)** has been linked to a reduction in both inflammatory and neuropathic pain, and has been shown to be beneficial for decreasing pain associated with rheumatoid arthritis, dysmenorrhea (pain during menstruation), inflammatory bowel disease, and neuropathy (Tokuyama 2011). Conversely, excessive levels of omega-6 PUFAs (found mostly in vegetable oils), such as arachidonic acid, are associated with inflammatory activities, an effect that can be offset by the simultaneous consumption of omega-3 PUFAs (Surette 2008). Every cell in the body has a bilayer phospholipid membrane wrapped around it to keep it protected — two layers of fat that keep the outside out and the inside in. These layers often become damaged and need repaired. If not, they produce the inflammation oxidation cycle and the pain continues. EFA's are what the body uses to repair them. Fish oils, flax seed oils, olive and coconut oils are the most commonly used oils, but there are three other oils that people should be aware of that work great as an antimicrobial, anti-inflammatory, and antioxidant oil.

Anti-inflammatory Oils

Chia *(Salvia hispanica L)* is a tropical and subtropical climates herbaceas plant from the mint family *(Lamiaceae)* which produces tiny, flavorless and white or dark brown seeds. Chia seeds have oval shape with approximately 1.9 - 2 mm long, 1 - 1.4 mm wide and 0.8 - 1 mm thickness diameter.[10]

Chia seed oil is extracted from the seeds and has been shown to be quite effective in producing health benefits ranging from reducing inflammation to fighting cancer.

Chia seeds are high in protein, fiber, and omega-3s, making them an excellent way to support metabolic health.

A study published in the journal, *Diabetes*, found that a diet high in monosaturated omega-9 fats, like the oil extracted from chia seeds, can reduce inflammation and improve insulin sensitivity.[11]

Chia seeds are rich in alpha lipoic acid (ALA) which is an omega-3 fatty acid.

In 2013, the *Journal of Molecular Biochemistry* found that ALA limited the growth of cancer cells in both breast and cervical cancers.

Researchers also found that it caused cell death of the cancer cells without harming the normal healthy cells. While more research still needs to be done to find out the deeper implications of ALA on other types of cancer, this is a great discovery for women struggling with these increasingly common types of cancer.[12]

Out of the several accompanying articles found in the tomb of Egyptian Pharaoh Tutankhamun were the seeds of black cumin *(Nigella sativa)*.[13] Not to be mistaken with common cumin seed *(Cuminum cyminum)*, it is a spice that grows in the Mediterranean region in western Asian countries including India, Pakistan, and Afghanistan. The historical references to these seeds are also found in some of the oldest religious and medical texts. For example, it is referred to as 'Melanthion' by Hippocrates and Dioscorides, while the Bible describes it as 'curative black cumin' (Isaiah 28:25, 27 NKJV).

Black cumin seed *(Nigella sativa)* oil extracts have been used for many centuries for the treatment of many human illnesses, and more recently the active compound found in black seed oil, viz. thymoquinone (TQ) has been tested for its efficacy against several diseases including cancer. The TQ extracted from the black cumin seeds are shown to have a significant antioxidant role and improves body's defense system, reduces apoptosis, and controls Akt pathway. Although the anti-cancer activity of *N. sativa* components was recognized thousands of years ago, but proper scientific research with this important traditional medicine is a history of the last 2-3 decades.[14]

In February 1995, doctors at the King's College London, U.K., tested black seed oil use for rheumatism and inflammatory diseases.[15]

In 1960, Professor El-Dakhakny reported that black seed oil has an anti-inflammatory effect and that it could be useful for relieving the effects of arthritis.

In 2002, at the Alexandria Medical Faculty, Alexandria, Egypt, he also studied the effectiveness of nigellone and thymoquinone whereby his research partly explained the mode of action of black seed's volatile oils in ameliorating inflammatory diseases.[16]

Palm oil is one of the few fatty fruits in existence; its likely to hold a substantial place in the human diet and is the second most consumed vegetable oil in the world.

It is different from other plant and animal oils in it's fatty acid composition (50% saturated, 40% unsaturated and 10% polyunsaturated).[17] In one study published in the *British Journal of Biomedical Science*, it was reported that despite the high levels of saturated fat in palm oil, the oil did not contribute to atherosclerosis or arterial thrombosis.[18] But in addition to MCFAs, palm oil is also enriched with the following phytonutrients: carotenoids (alpha-beta-and gamma-carotenes), steroids (sitosterol, stigmasterol, and campesterol), water-soluble powerful antioxidants, phenolic compounds, and flavonoids.

Tocotrienol and tocopherol make up 70% to 30% of the vit E present in red palm oil respectively.[19] The tocotrienols have been suggested to inhibit HMG-CoA reductase enzyme activity and thus regulate serum cholesterols.[20]

Arthritis is an inflammatory joint disease that results in destruction of the articular cartilage.

In one specific study, palm tocotrienol fractions from palm oil have been shown to possess anti-inflammatory effects and provide (a potential) a new nutrient for reducing arthritis. The results of this study revealed that the use of palm oil tocotrienols significantly down regulated the production of COX-2 inflammatory enzymes, IL-b, IL-6 and MMP-3 in arthritis.

In addition, palm tocotrienol fraction induced TIMPs that produce anti-inflammatory effect to block inflammation directly in arthritis. These findings show that palm tocotrienol fractions may be of potential therapeutic value in regulating the joint destruction in arthritis.[21]

Plant-based oils are readily available and research has shown they can have significant effects on blocking inflammatory processes as well as enhancing immune function. Although there is a lack of studies showing the effect of all three of those plant based oils used together, and demonstrating their combined effects, it stands to reason that the cumulative effects would provide profound health benefits for those who consume them.

L-lysine is most popularly known as the antiviral that stops progression of the herpes simplex virus that causes fever blisters. If you take L-lysine before the blister breaks out, it can stop the replication of the virus and will stop it in its tracks. A typical dose for this would be about 1000-1500 mg per day. When you increase the dosage to around 3000 mg per day, something amazing happens. Remember all of those billiard balls that get jammed underneath the blood vessel linings and turn into foam cells that narrow your vessels (atherosclerosis)? The Linus Pauling Institute published a study showing that L-lysine actually draws out those billiard balls and foam cells from those vessels when used for a length of time.

Instead of waiting until it is time to have a stent, why not start working on it now before the vessel gets closed up? A good preventative might be to put 3,000 mg of L-lysine into your body daily to help prevent this from happening.

Vitamin D, specifically vitamin D3, has most recently been popularized based on new clinical research revealing the many health benefits it possesses. Most people already know **vitamin D** helps you to absorb calcium. However, research has revealed another very important benefit of this powerful antioxidant. Studies show that adequate levels of vitamin D lead to less inflammation and lower levels of inflammatory cytokines and prostaglandins.[22] Indeed, vitamin D deficiency has been reported as a risk factor for different forms of inflammatory diseases.[23] This is such a valuable asset for chronic pain sufferers because based on the research, supplementing with vitamin D can improve the inflammation that's causing people to suffer with pain. Chronic inflammation affects everything in the body and can have a significant effect on the metabolism. What most people do not know is that vitamin D also helps you metabolize fat. In the *Nutrition Journal* [2013], a research study was done where they combined vitamin D with a very small dose of calcium. They took fifty-three subjects that were college students. They instructed those college students to continue with their usual unhealthy eating habits. The only thing they allowed them to do different is they gave them a very low dosage of calcium along with some vitamin D3. They did this for twelve weeks, and the conclusion was simply this: Upon the D3 supplementation for twelve weeks, it augmented body fat and visceral fat loss significantly.[24] What does that mean? That means the weight around the belly came off just from adding D3 and a little bit of calcium to the diet. It is amazing how effective nutrients like vitamin D can be for reducing inflammation, relieving pain, and affecting weight loss and metabolism.

There is a vitamin D3 craze out right now; again, you have to watch the fads. I am trying to warn you. The current fad is instructing everyone that is deficient in vitamin D to get their blood levels up to over 70, even as high as 100. Clinically this may be appropriate for people with certain disorders, or severe deficiencies, and especially for those who have had severe long-term conditions who are trying to recover that requires these doses. However, the bell curves from the most reliable and extensive studies clearly show the optimal "maintenance levels" to fall between 35-40. It's important to remember when you look at vitamin D levels, the focus shouldn't be only on correcting the deficient level. This, along with all deficiencies is the wrong approach. If you step back and look at the big picture, there's usually a more systemic reason for the deficiency to be present. Certainly, the deficient levels need to be supplemented to raise them, but the cause should also be investigated as well. Example, I have found in my own clinical experience, that many people with problems with their fat metabolisms, especially people with an underactive thyroid, have vitamin D deficiency. Vitamin D is a fat-soluble vitamin. If you don't help correct the body's ability to digest and assimilate fats properly, then that person will have to take supplementation from now on because they can't utilize the vitamin from their diet. I usually always recommend a bioemulsified form, which means it's already broken down, until both the fat digestion and assimilation problem, along with the deficiency problem, are all corrected.

Most studies agree, that even when a deficiency was present, not to exceed more than about ten thousand units daily to reestablish adequate levels. Doctors in the U.S. often prescribe Drisdol (vitamin D2) for vitamin D deficiency, giving 50,000 IU every week or two for 8-12 weeks. Then, a few give it every month. Too many forget about their patient's vitamin D deficiency, thinking the Drisdol has cured it forever. There are two problems with this approach:

First, Drisdol is not human vitamin D.

Secondly, the same habits that caused the vitamin D deficiency in the first place continue, and cause deficiency again, eventually, after treatment finishes. The dosage prescribed in this protocol can also be problematic because it can produce some scary side effects for the patient consuming it. I've had patients report to me that their hearts were pounding and that they had a great deal of anxiety taking that prescribed dose. Some have reported nausea and a general feeling that something was not right in their system. Personally I have never clinically had any condition where I had to administer vitamin D (vitamin D3) in that high of dose. Quite frequently patient's vitamin D levels are in the low twenties and are raised in the eighties and sometimes as high as a hundred in chronic degenerative states, but it's never taken more than ten thousand daily to raise those levels. Dr. Victoria Logan and colleagues of the University of Otago in New Zealand have added yet another reason why Drisdol should not be prescribed. In a recent study, they have shown that not only is vitamin D2 less effective in raising 25(OH)D levels than vitamin D3, but that Drisdol actually lowers 25(OH)D3 levels. That is, when 25(OH)D2 is present in the blood, 25(OH)D3 levels go down.[25] The obvious takeaway message is, "Don't take a supplement that causes a deficiency, especially when it's supposed to correct the deficiency you already have." Adequate doses of K2 sometimes need to be administered along with the vitamin D if the levels do not improve with supplementation and dietary recommendations.

One of the most impressive things I personally have observed about vitamin D clinically is when someone is deficient and those levels are restored, all types of pain syndromes are resolved as well.

Once a person gains control of the chronic oxidative and inflammatory processes in their body, they can actually move better, feel better, and have more energy. The tissues then can begin to repair allowing structures to heal. This enables that person to have the ability to do things they could not do before. People that have not been able to do activities for years are able to go out and do them. The more activity they do, the more they can do: and more breeds more. It initiates an entire cycle of healing. It breaks them out of that downward spiral of disease and pain, reversing the process, allowing them to recover.

Conclusion

The entire body from the cardiovascular system, to the brain, to all of the organ systems, and all of the vital structures, all of them are affected by oxidation and inflammation. The top killers in America are heart disease, cancer, strokes, atherosclerosis, and diabetes; all of these conditions involve oxidation and inflammation in their etiology. These processes continue to break down the tissues and linings causing severe degenerative and conditions. These degenerative processes continue to progress over time and produce even more cellular damage and tissue destruction until eventually they end up causing intense, severe, overwhelming and sometimes debilitating pain. By reducing the oxidation and inflammation these conditions can start to improve, radically reducing, or in most cases, eliminating the severe pain. The takeaway message is simply this: Stop the oxidation and inflammation = STOP THE PAIN.

> **Stop the oxidation and inflammation = STOP THE PAIN.**

Chapter 5: Stop the Oxidation

1. Dramatic lowering of very high Lp(a) in response to niacin Min Li, MD, PhD, Ramesh Saeedi, MD, PhD, Simon W. Rabkin, MD, Jiri Frohlich, MD, Email the author MD Jiri Frohlich Healthy Heart Program Prevention Clinic, St. Paul's Hospital, Vancouver, BC, Canada Published Online: March 29, 2014.

2. High Exposure to Radio Frequency Radiation Associated with Cancer in Male Rats News Release; NIEHS; For Immediate Release Thursday, November 1, 2018, 10:00 a.m. EDT.

3. Effects of electromagnetic fields exposure on the antioxidant defense system Elfide Gizem Kıvrak, Kıymet Kübra Yurt, [...], and Gamze Altun J Microsc Ultrastruct. 2017 Oct-Dec :5(4):167-176.

4. Advanced Glycation End Products in Foods and a Practical Guide to Their Reduction in the Diet JAIME URIBARRI, MD, SANDRA WOODRUFF, RD, [...], and HELEN VLASSARA, MD J Am. Diet Assoc. 2010 Jun :110(6):911-16.e.12.

5. Advanced Glycation End Products Sparking the Development of Diabetic Vascular Injury Alison Goldin, Joshua A. Beckman, Ann Marie Schmidt, and Mark A. Creager. Originally published 8 Aug 2006 Circulation. 2006;114:597–605.

6. J Soc Biol. 2001;195(4):387-90. [Advanced glycation end products (AGEs), free radicals and diabetes]. [Article in French] Gillery P1. Dietary Advanced Glycation End Products and Their Role in Health and Disease.

7. Jaime Uribarri, María Dolores del Castillo, María Pía de la Maza, Rosana Filip, Alejandro Gugliucci, Claudia Luevano-Contreras, Maciste H Macías-Cervantes, Deborah H Markowicz, Bastos Alejandra Medrano, Teresita Menini... Show more Advances in Nutrition, Volume 6, Issue 4, 1 July 2015, Pages 461–473, https://doi.org/10.3945/an.115.008433 Published: 07 July 2015.

8. Dr.Hans Napier, Townsend Letter to Doctors and Patients; April 1997 issue.

9. Nicer Assyrian. Faris Nasser and Maria Grosovski; Olive oil consumption and non-alcoholic fatty acid liver disease; world Gastroenterol. 2009 Apr 21;15(15) :1809-1815.

10. Ixtaina V.Y., Nolasco S.M., Tomas M.C. "Physical Properties of Chia (Saliva hispanica L) seeds." *Ind crop Prod.* 2008; 28:286-93.

11. "Monounsaturated fatty acid-enriched high fat diets impeded adipose NLRP3 inflammasome-mediated IL-Ib secretion and insulin resistance despite obesity." Diabetes. 2015 Jun; 64 (6): 2116-28.

12. Rashmi Deshpande, Prakash Mansara, Srehal Suryavan Ruchka Kaul-Ghanekar, "Alpha-Imolenic acid regulates the growth of breast and cervical cancer cell: lines through regulation of NO release and induction of lipid peroxidase. The author(s) 2013. Published by Lorom Ipsum Press. *Journal of Molecular Biochemistry* (2013) 2, 6-17.

13. Nigella Sativa; (Zohary and Hopt, 2001).

14. Asaduzzaman Khan, Han-chun Chen, [m], and Dian-zheng Zhang. "Anticancer Activities of *Nigella Sativa* (Black Cumin), *African Journal of Traditional, Complementary and Alternative Medicines:AJTCAM*, 2011:8 (5 Suppl): 226-232.

15. Houghton PJ1, Zarka R, de las Heras B, Hoult JR. "Fixed oil of Nigella sativa and derived thymoquinone inhibit eicosanoid gereration in leukocytes and membrane lipid peroxidation." Planta Med. 1995 Feb;61(1):33-6.

16. El-Dakhakhny M', Madi N.J., Lembert N, T Ammon H.P. "*Nigella sativa* oil, nigellone and derived thymoquinone to inhibit synthesis of 5-lipoxygenase products in polymorphonclear leukocytes from rats." *J Ethnopharmacol.* 2002 July, 81 (2): 161-4.

17. Boyle & Anderson, Thomson/Wadsworth. Personal Nutrition, 6th ed., 2007.

18. Oguntibeju, Esterhuyse A.J, Truter E.J. "Red palm oil: Nutritional, physiological and therapeutic roles in improving human well-being and quality of life." *B.J. Biomed Sci* 2009;66 (4). 216-22.

19. Sambanthamurthi R, Sundram K, Tan Y. "Chemistry and biochemistry of palm oil." *Prog Lipid Res.* 2000; 39: 507-558. [Pub Med] [Refl List].

20. Sundram K., Sambanthamurthi R., Tan YA. "Palm fruit chemistry and nutrition." *Asia Pac J Clin Nutr.* 2003, 12:355-362 [Pub Med] [Ref List].

21. Zainal Z., Abdul Hafrid and Shahrin Z. (2013). "Anti-inflammatory effect of palm oil tocotrienol fractions on arthritis." Front. Immonol. Conference abstract: 15 International Congress of Immunology (ICI), doi: 10,3389/conf.fimmu. 2013. 02.01198.

22. Gendelman O., itzhaki D., Makarov S., Bennun M, Amital H. A randomized double-blind placebo-controlled study adding high dose vitamin D to analgesic regimens in patients with musculoskeletal pain. Lupus. 2015;24:483-489.

23. Gatenby P., Lucas R., Swamnathan A., Vitamin D deficiency and risk for rheumatic diseases: An update.Curr. Opin. Rheumatol. 2013;25:184-191.doi:10:1097/BOR.0b013e32835cfc16 [pubmed] Lee Y.H., Bae S.C. Vitamin D level in rheumatoid arthritis and its correlation with the disease activity.;A meta-analysis .Clin. Exp. Rheumatol.2016;34:827-833 [pubmed].

24. The beneficial role of vitamin D in obesity: possible genetic and cell signaling mechanisms. Khanh vinh quốc Lương and Lan Thi Hoàng Nguyễn ; Nutr J 2013;12;89.

25. Logan VF, Gray AR, Peddie MC, Harper MJ, Houghton LA. Long-term vitamin D3 supplementation is more effective than vitamin D2 in maintaining serum 25-hydroxyvitamin D status over the winter months. Br J Nutr. 2012 Jul 11:1-7.

CHAPTER SIX

Balancing the Gut
Fiber Forever

The colon is like a big dumpster where the unusable items accumulate and are stored until it is convenient to expel its content. When the diet has plenty of fiber, the debris gets swept away. Like a big mop, the fiber grabs everything, and sticks to it, and it pulls it through the colon. Then it pushes it out for safe evacuation. We call this process a bowel movement (BM).

Just as digestion is important, good bowel habits are essential for good health and especially beneficial for removing the harmful toxins that, if accumulated in the system, can cause damage leading to significant pain and discomfort. Remember, when you eat food, it is supposed to be used for fuel, but you have to understand that food is foreign to the body. It is not part of the natural body. So every time food comes in, it has to be vetted and pass inspection and an acceptance process that the body puts it through to make sure that it can stay and be utilized. All substances that enter into the body in any way also have to go through the same vetting process. If food is present and does not pass inspection, the defense systems release inflammatory cytokines in response. This causes the body to inflame and the viscous cycle of pain begins and will continually repeat itself. Food needs to be digested and its wastes eliminated. If anything impairs this process, systemic disruptions, symptoms, pain, and inflammation will most likely be the result.

Fiber is so important because it helps to prevent foods from staying in the gut too long. Psyllium fiber is a very good insoluble fiber because it accomplishes the task of being a bulking agent to cleanse the bowel, but has a very low probability of causing a gut sensitivity reaction. One of the very first things I do with my patients who have chronic pain syndromes is to work on developing good bowel habits. Two to three bowel movements a day is a good baseline normal. The buildup of toxins in the body can damage cells causing inflammation, pain, and produce a host of bad symptoms throughout the body. Poor elimination and assimilation is what causes theses toxins to back up and build up. Many times I have asked patients if they were constipated and they would tell me they were not. Then I would ask them how many bowel movements they had each day and they would tell me they had one every couple of days. The sad thing is, they thought that was normal. When they would ask me what normal was, I would answer them with a question. "How many times do you eat each day? Three times? Think of it as being like a Play-Doh Factory, something in--something out. Got it?"

> **Two to three bowel movements a day is a good baseline normal.**

The correct answer should have been, "How many times do you eat each day?" "Three times!" "How many times do you have a bowel movement each day?" "Three times." It's pretty simple, right? Nature's pharmacy is full of natural substances that assist the body with proper elimination and assimilation. Fresh fruits and vegetables are loaded with fiber content and are an excellent choice for promoting elimination. When most people think of fiber they think of wheat-based grains. The problem with wheat products is that many of them are genetically modified and produce sensitivity reactions in the gut. This can actually add to the problem of elimination instead of improve it. Oats have a time-tested record for being a quality fiber, but certain people may still have a cross-reactive sensitivity to gluten if they consume them. Fruits and vegetables still contain the best fibers for the gut in my opinion, especially when someone is inflamed and is eliminating grains from the diet. Psyllium husks are also a good option.

Another important aspect of promoting good bowel function is hydrating the bowel. Drink plenty of filtered water, at least several twelve-ounce glasses each day. Drink it about 30 minutes before you eat a meal and it can actually help you to eat less by reducing cravings and making you full faster. There are many times when someone is partially dehydrated and is thirsty, yet interprets that as hunger and looks to food to fix the problem. For a really nice boost, a couple of times each day add a fat sprinkle of pink Himalayan salts, a drop or two of ginger oil, and a little stevia extract, squeeze half of a lemon, and mix it all together in a glass of water. It does wonders for improving gut transient time and helps improve bowel function. Taking some extra magnesium and some vitamin C can be helpful when the bowels have been stressed and acts as a mild cathartic by relaxing the bowel to promote a smooth painless bowel movement. A nice hot cup of organic coffee or tea also gets that bowel moving. One of the most important things you can do to stimulate bowel activity is "movement." Get out there and start walking, riding a bike, or doing some form of exercise every day. If you are not having the normal number of BMs each day, your colon is probably backing up toxins in the system. I actually have normal bowel function but still supplement with fiber and follow this same **advice** daily because I want to do whatever is necessary to make sure these toxins don't back up and cause harm to my body. It's so important to do the things that are necessary to prevent these toxins from building up and causing damage to our systems.

The Microbiome

The cells in certain parts of the lining of the digestive tract are actually as thin as onionskin. This causes the gut to be extremely sensitive. Other portions are much thicker, like when we get down to the more transient parts of the intestine. Along the intestines, there are little villi and hair-like processes that help food move along through the process of **peristalsis**; there is a whole ecological system in your bowel. The comprehensive term is referred to as the **microbiome** of the gut. There are roughly between 300-1000 different species of microorganisms living there. There are good bugs and bad bugs. There are good yeast and bad yeast. There are good bacteria and bad bacteria. The good, normal bacteria are called **intestinal flora**. They live in your gut and coexist with the yeast to create a balance in the microbiome. They are also one of the first lines of defense in the body.

Sometimes we consume things that wreak havoc in the bowel, things like antibiotics. When you take antibiotics, they wipe out most everything — the good, the bad, and the ugly. The problem is, they do not affect the yeast. The gut has to have the right balance of intestinal flora to yeast ratio. It is like the Hatfields and the Mc-Coys. As long as there are enough Hatfields, there are not too many McCoys and as long as there are enough McCoys, there are not too many Hatfields. They keep each other in check. Nobody really gains

any ground. Everybody just stays in check. However, if you get rid
of all the Hatfields, guess who takes over? The McCoys. So if an
antibiotic, chlorinated water, or some other toxic substance destroys
a large population of the bacteria, guess who takes over the gut? The
yeast! These yeast can proliferate in your gut, migrate through the
epithelial linings and cause an imbalance called **intestinal dysbiosis**.
They can even spread to the urinary tract and cause infection there
as well. Yeast can be very destructive when they are out of balance
and can be difficult to manage if left in this state for long periods
of time. Often, if left untreated, they are capable of provoking a lot
of inflammatory responses in the endothelial lining of the gut and
also depositing toxic residues called **mycotoxins**. These substances
are quite toxic and can lead to sickness and disease. Anytime the
bowel is inflamed it is quite common for inflammatory cytokines
to be released into the peripheral system causing pain, joint swelling, muscle soreness, headaches, and even sinus pain and congestion. Most people who suffer with these symptoms never even
consider this kind of gut imbalance to be the root cause of their
pain and suffering. The really sad part is, neither do some of their
doctors. Those suffering from the overpopulation of yeast usually have excessive cravings especially for sugar. Once the sugar is
consumed the yeast feast. It's equivalent to leaving candy outside on
the ground. It doesn't take long and it will be covered in bugs. Sugar
fuels yeast like gas fuels fire; it sends them out of control. Whether
it be **candida** or any other strain of yeast, once the imbalance occurs
they can wreak havoc on the body. From excessive fatigue to severe
systemic pain, these yeast overgrowths can cause some pretty nasty
symptoms. When they spin out of control they must be put back
in their normal balance or the person suffering will not be able to
regain control of their health. Nature's pharmacy provides many
substances that can help to eliminate this imbalance. Oregano oil,

caprylic acid, olive leaf extract, and of course probiotics, are just a few of many natural substances that research suggests can be highly effective against these yeast. BIOCLEANSE has these as well as a comprehensive formulation to help restore things back to normal. This process usually takes about 3-6 months to bring back to balance. Completely eliminating sugar, refined carbs, and all fruits, are imperative through this time frame. Remember, the dietary restrictions listed for each condition in this book are temporary and are necessary for complete recovery. You will be able to add these foods back after the process is complete in most cases.

Infectious microorganisms can also enter the gut and cause it to inflame. **Parasites** from undercooked, contaminated, or poorly prepared food quite commonly are the culprits of such infections. **Gram-negative bacteria** are also notorious bad bugs in the gut. These all have the potential to cause infection, irritation, inflammation, and even death if left untreated. They are capable of creating extensive damage to the gut and its related organs. If left undetected and untreated they can cause crippling and debilitating effects in the body that can also be accompanied by excessive pain.

I had a patient many years ago that came to see me who was in a wheelchair. A few months before he was a healthy, normal evangelist who was out teaching and preaching while keeping a rigorous schedule. He went on a mission trip overseas and when he returned to the states, his health suddenly nosedived. He started having intense back pain that radiated down his leg. He could not remember falling or straining it, but the pain was getting more and more severe each day. He went to see his physician who immediately put him on pain medications and muscle relaxers. The pain was some better as long as he was taking the medication, but if he was ever late taking it, the intense pain would return. As time went on, the pain also migrated into both legs until finally he was unable to walk on them at all, confining him to a wheelchair. That's the point when he consulted me.

On the initial visit while taking his history, he was telling me about his missions trip overseas. I interrupted him in the middle of his story and asked if he had eaten anything different than his usual diet while over there. He could not think of anything at that moment. I then asked if he had any shellfish while he was out of the country and his entire countenance changed. He suddenly remembered that the night before he left, he ate raw oysters and recalled it was the first time in years that he had eaten them. Bingo! I felt I knew exactly what was going on. I ran some tests that confirmed my suspicion and started treating him for a parasite using high potency standardized herbal extracts and nutraceuticals. Within one week his pain was almost gone and by the end of the second week, he was able to get out of his wheelchair unassisted. After a few weeks he regained all of the strength in his legs and was back to his normal self. Not every case responds this dramatically, but many of them do. When you find the correct cause and use the right treatment, the results are usually nothing short of miraculous. Think about it for a moment; a man in a wheelchair with debilitating pain resolved by killing a parasite using nature's pharmacy. When people have been to all of the specialists and they are no better or even worse, they may have to take a different approach and look at things in a new and different way, if they ever want to fully recover and STOP THE PAIN.

There are a lot of people who get stomachaches, vomiting, diarrhea, cramping, and even abdominal pain shortly after they eat a meal and just suffer through it. What most people don't realize is that if they would take a few probiotics immediately following the questionable meal, they could probably resolve the problem before it manifests as the painful symptoms. Just the other day I was on the way to play tennis with my son. We had just eaten at a restaurant where I had a bowl of cole slaw with my meal. We had only been gone from the restaurant for about 5 minutes and I felt my throat starting to tighten up with a slight sore throat. Most people would think the problem was probably just something that was going around and feel that maybe someone had coughed on them that day or that they came in contact with someone sick. The truth is, I knew exactly what was wrong. Something was wrong with that cole slaw I had eaten. I immediately went by my house on the way to the courts to get some probiotic capsules. By the time I pulled into the driveway I had already started feeling slight flu symptoms. I swallowed several of the probiotics capsules and headed for the courts. When we arrived at the tennis courts, about ten minutes away, my symptoms were completely gone and I played with my normal energy and had no more symptoms as a result.

> **Anytime you watch a commercial on TV with five seconds of benefits from a wonderful new wonder drug, and forty-five seconds of side effects from the damage it causes in your system, this should be convincing enough.**

There have been so many occasions when I have instructed my family, friends, and patients to take some probiotics following a questionable meal and it saved them from getting a host of symptoms that probably would get blamed on the flu or a stomach virus. If you are ever finishing a meal and suddenly start to feel symptoms, don't wait; take some probiotics. You also have to watch for undercooked foods. If you are eating a meal and realize that the meat is undercooked, you may also want to take a few digestive enzymes as well. This will assist in destroying microbes or parasites that may be present. Many of the symptoms that people experience after eating bad food manifest as flu symptoms, coughing, congestion, a scratchy and/ or sore throat. They are not caused from cold, flu, or viruses but instead they are caused by mild forms of dysentery (gut bugs). When someone has symptoms after eating that are caused from "gut bugs," probiotics can make the difference in a lot of these cases.

What else destroys the gut lining? Alcohol, drugs, prescription or nonprescription medications can damage these linings. Use common sense; Anytime you watch a commercial on TV with five seconds of benefits from a wonderful new wonder drug, and forty-five seconds of side effects from the damage it causes in your system, this should be convincing enough. Before we put anything in our mouths, we need to consider if the benefit outweighs the potential consequences. Many of these highly advertised drugs could cause a lot of damage to the gut linings.

Too Much of a Good Thing Can Be a Bad Thing

Probiotics have recently been glamorized as being the holy grail for gut problems. This may, in fact, be true in many cases, but like anything else, balance is the key. Due to their popularity and easy availability, they are being consumed in record quantities. People are loading up on probiotics and even taking excessively high doses. Remember the Hatfield's and McCoy's talk? If you have too many of one, they will take over. After completing a round of antibiotics, it makes sense to take a reasonable dose to reestablish a healthy balance. New research suggests that it may actually take up to one year to reestablish that balance. Once they repopulate the bowel, the yeast are put back in check and everything goes back to normal. The problem starts when the shift swings the other way. When some-

❝ Q: What is the best plan to help you recover and STOP THE PAIN?

A: THE ONE YOU WILL DO!❞

one takes too many probiotics or disturbs the normal balance, the bacteria take over and cause problems of their own. This condition is called **Small Intestinal Bacterial Overgrowth syndrome (SIBO)** and once this condition manifests, it needs to be corrected by repopulating the gut with the correct balance of yeast. **Saccharomyces Boulardii** is the most common yeast used as a supplement in order to reestablish this balance and reverse the SIBO. There are simple saliva and even breath tests that can be used to find out if someone is out of balance or not. If you have had a chronic gut problem that has not been responding to treatment, you may want to have this tested.

The Road to Recovery Can Be Quite Simple in Concept:

1. Take out the foods that are offending, put in the substances that promote healing.

2. Stay away from drugs that have harmful side effects in order to prevent damaging cells further.

3. Make a conscious effort to determine the imbalances in the body using whatever tests or exams are needed.

4. Establish a strategy that includes a plan for making lifestyle changes while correcting the deficiencies and imbalances that the tests and exams reveal.

5. Do not deviate from the plan unless instructed by a health professional .

QUESTION:

What is the best plan to help you recover and STOP THE PAIN?

ANSWER:

"THE ONE YOU WILL DO!"
Be consistent and stay committed.

 If someone's gut has been really messed up for a long time, it may take, on the average, about six months or more to heal. Do not expect for all of the symptoms to go away immediately. That is an unreasonable expectation, especially for chronic conditions. The damage that took years to create may take a few months, and in some cases, a couple of years to heal. Of course certain cases respond immediately and symptoms may disappear rapidly, but that doesn't mean that the problem is gone. The gut needs to be treated and monitored until the imbalances are corrected. The symptoms don't dictate whether the treatment is working or not. In fact, sometimes the patient's symptoms get worse when they start treatment because of the rapid die off of microorganisms and the toxic residues they leave behind. This is called a **Herxheimer reaction**. Be persistent, stay consistent, and don't stop doing what's fixing the problem just because you feel better.

Dead Food

Can you imagine someone going to a restaurant and telling the waiter to bring them a large order of **dead food** that has had its vital nutrients and enzymes destroyed? That's exactly what people do every day when they eat foods out of bags, boxes, and packages. The food is dead and depleted. It doesn't have the enzymes and nutrients that it had when it was still alive. When raw foods are eaten they have life inside of the cells of that food. The food is jam-packed full of energy-producing substances that add life back to a tired body. Some folks love to cook foods "to death," destroying all of the components that bring vitality to the system. Sometimes it's cooked so much that it cannot be recognized by its look or taste.

It's nice when the vegetable is the same color as it was in the garden when it's eaten. When the food is alive, the enzymes and the fibers are preserved in the food. This helps the digestion and absorption in the gut while it also encourages the bowel to evacuate properly. These foods do not steal energy but instead provide it. Everyone should incorporate some raw foods into the diet every day. You should be eating some raw foods at least a couple of times a day. I am not instructing anyone to turn into a rabbit, but I am saying you need to incorporate plenty of raw foods into your diet. Of course organic foods are much healthier, but in most cases they are too expensive or hard to get. Nonorganic foods will suffice but make sure you wash your foods well. That's at least a good preventative measure. You've probably heard some of these recommendations many times in the past, but are you doing them? Start today. Keep a diet journal so you can actually record how much raw food content you are really eating. If you don't do it today, this way, then you probably won't do it at all. "Stop making excuses and start making progress."

> " Stop making excuses and start making progress. "

CHAPTER SEVEN

Antioxidant Systems and Nutrients

Vitamin, Minerals, and Plant Antioxidants

Vitamin A, especially in the form of beta-carotene, is a great antioxidant for the eyes and skin. A deficiency of vitamin A can be one of the reasons people may suffer from night blindness. This is a condition that makes it very difficult to see while driving at night because the eyes become extremely sensitive to oncoming headlights. Vitamin A is a fat-soluble vitamin and can reach a toxic level in the body if too much is consumed. Beta-carotene is water-soluble and can be consumed long term and at much higher doses with no known side effects. The body will convert it into vitamin A, and any excess will pass through the urine before it builds up any toxicity. That is why beta-carotene is a very popular antioxidant. Both vitamin A and beta-carotene are powerful antioxidants but also are a good adjunct for boosting the immune system.

Vitamin C is one of the most useful antioxidants on the planet.

Research supports health benefits ranging from boosting immunity, healing and repairing tissues, to claims of antiaging, cancer prevention, and a long distinguished list of other uses. There are multiple studies that have been done on vitamin C that have shown that it can stimulate the production of collagen and proteoglycan (both of which are important parts of joint cartilage) and can protect against the breakdown of cartilage in animal studies. It would take another entire book to adequately explain all of the health benefits this nutrient delivers. The obvious conclusion here is you need to take vitamin C. One commonly asked question is, "How do I know how much vitamin C I need?" A very simple way to saturate your system to make sure your levels are at full capacity is to start taking vitamin C at a dose one gram (1000 mg) every two hours, and continue taking until your stool becomes loose. If you start to get diarrhea or symptoms of a loose stool, stop. You are at saturation. Then do a

"One of the most beneficial uses that most people are not aware of is the effect vitamin E has on chronic arthritis."

maintenance dose, maybe a couple of grams or slightly more a day to maintain that level. Sometimes it takes a few days to reach saturation in those who are severely depleted.

Vitamin C is typically a safe antioxidant for most people; however, if taken in higher doses, especially in an IV, **a glucose-6-phosphate dehydrogenase blood test** should be performed. If this enzyme is deficient, there is probably a genetic factor that prevents the proper breakdown and assimilation of the vitamin C and can cause serious and potentially fatal side effects.

Vitamin E is another powerful antioxidant, especially for the cardiovascular system. Some studies have shown not to take over four hundred units a day. Some studies show that you can take up to a thousand. You should be safe as long as you stay in that range from 400 to 1000 IU. The best and most complete form of vitamin E is called mixed tocopherols. This antioxidant is one of the most cardioprotective antioxidants of its kind. When mixed with selenium the antioxidant effect is even more powerful.

One of the most beneficial uses that most people are not aware of is the effect vitamin E has on chronic arthritis. Clinical signs and symptoms of osteoarthritis include pain, stiffness, restricted motion, and crepitus. It is the major cause of joint dysfunction in developed nations and has enormous social and economic consequences. Current treatments focus on symptomatic relief; however, they lack efficacy in controlling the progression of this disease, which is a leading cause of disability. Vitamin E is safe to use and may delay the progression of osteoarthritis by acting on several aspects of the disease.[1] This is certainly a safer approach for people who suffer from arthritis.

Vitamins A, C, and E have powerful antioxidant properties and have been used safely for many years as supplemental vitamins. This means they can override harmful free radicals which are produced within your cells that cause tissue damage or disease. Your body produces its own antioxidants but research suggests that antioxidants in the diet help destroy excess free radicals that produce the damage that lead to pain and suffering.

No one should ever take a megadose of any nutrient unless they are being tested and monitored by a licensed physician. Each one of these nutrients has a toleration limitation that your body can metabolize at any one time. If you try to exceed that, it can cause serious toxic reactions and extensive cell damage. However, when you are going through periods when you are experiencing higher levels of stress you may want to ramp up the antioxidants a bit. The most important part of antioxidant therapy is to stay diligent and not be complacent. Everybody is well meaning and they start out doing pretty good, but sometimes they do not always follow through on their supplementation like they should. There are certainly more vitamin antioxidants than are listed here, but these are the ones that apply the most to the subject matter.

Mineral Antioxidants

There are a host of mineral antioxidants. Zinc, selenium, manganese, molybdenum, and magnesium, etc. are all excellent antioxidants. They also serve as catalysts for all kind of functions in the body from hair growth to detoxification and are vital for growth, repair, energy production, elimination, and other critical functions in the body. Mineral supplementation is an essential part most every form of recovery program from chronic gut problems to long-term addictions. Minerals help the body to recover from damage and can be very beneficial in the elimination of pain. From energy production to systemic detoxification, minerals are vital for the normal function of these processes.

Plant-based Antioxidants
Ellagitannins

Some of the strongest antioxidants available come from plants. Many of these compounds are used by clinicians to treat a variety of conditions. When used in this capacity they are commonly referred to as nutraceuticals. There are many of these natural antioxidants that have tremendous medicinal value as well. One group in particular has shown much promise in the prevention and reduction of sickness and disease, especially the ones extracted from red raspberry. These powerful phenol antioxidants have been shown by research studies to improve circulation, alleviate muscle fatigue and soreness, stave off infections, and support immune function, benefits the digestive tract and even promotes healthy skin. **Ellagitannins** in particular are specific phenols that can provide significant health benefits. The reason why I like ellagitannins so much is because, for the most part, they are well tolerated and they help stop oxidation that weakens the immune system and destroys cells. When something damages cells the DNA gets disrupted. This can cause those cells to begin expressing abnormally and can ultimately end up producing cancer cells. When someone consumes adequate doses of ellagitannins, it helps block and stop this process as well as enhances the immune system.

Fungal infections and contamination of food products by these toxic microorganisms can play a huge role in immune activation. They can provoke cytokine responses that lead to inflammatory responses and even allergic responses in some cases. If left untreated they can cause prolonged immune responses that can lead to autoimmune diseases and can compromise the immune system. Many hidden sinus infections are caused from fungal invasion. A study published in June of 2013 evaluated the use of the ellagitannins from red raspberries used as an antifungal agent. The study demonstrated that ellagitannins obtained from red raspberry (Rubus idaeus L.) fruit exhibit in vitro and in situ antifungal activity.[2]

The pharmacological activities of tannins described in medicinal books before the recent achievements on ellagitannin chemistry were mostly those of gallotannins and condensed tannins of poor chemical uniformity.[3] The newer updated testing procedures are revealing new benefits that previously were not realized. As for ellagitannins, although some members of this class of hydrolyzable tannins were obtained early on, it is the isolation and structural determination of over 500 pure compounds since 1975 from various plants, many of which used in traditional medicines, that brought remarkable changes in the definition and concept of "tannins."[4] Researchers discovered that Helicobacter pylori (HP) was potently inhibited by these compounds. HP is a Gram-negative spirillum that may cause chronic gastritis, gastric ulcer, duodenal ulcer, and also stomach cancer. MRSA (methicillin-resistant Staphylo-coccus aureus) aquiring multi-drug resistance was restored by them as well. The more recent studies show that these powerful compounds also inhibit tumor formation in certain types of cancer[5] and induce apoptosis (cell death) in certain cancer cells.[6] The benefits were in part believed to have been as a result of the ellagitannins enhancing the immune response.[7] Ellagitannins are powerful antioxidants that according to research also have amazing immune enhancing effects, which are paramount in those who are having trouble recovering from illness. They also seem to be an obvious choice for the prevention of sickness and disease as well.

Spirulina is another popular plant antioxidant. It's also called super blue green algae. It has powerful antioxidant and anti-inflammatory properties that are well tolerated by the human body. Per 100 grams of Spirulina, 57.5 of those grams are protein which makes it one of the highest protein food sources. Pound for pound it has more protein than red meat! Vegetarians use this as an alternative source for protein.[8]

Spirulina can help boost aerobic performance as shown in a study done of nine moderately trained males. Each of them took either six grams per day of spirulina supplement or placebo for four weeks.

At the end of each two-hour run, exercise performance and respiratory quotient were tested for both placebo and spirulina. Subjects who took spirulina had better stamina (it took them longer to get fatigued) and had significantly lower carbohydrate oxidation rate compared to placebo.[9]

In 1988 the first clinical study was done on 30 healthy male subjects who had mild hyperlipidemia or hypertension. Half were given 4.2 grams spirulina every day for eight weeks, while the other half were given the same dose for four weeks.

Both groups ate the same thing for the next four weeks. After the study, both groups were able to lower their cholesterol levels significantly. However, when they stopped taking spirulina supplement, their cholesterol levels went back to the baseline. After the eight-week period, there was an increase in HDL levels (good cholesterol) by individuals who took spirulina supplement.

Type-2 Diabetics may want to consider spirulina as a supplement to help control blood sugar levels. In a study done to twenty-five people who have type-2 diabetes that were given two grams/day for two months resulted in the reduction of fasting and postprandial blood sugar levels.[10]

Research has shown that spirulina contains ingredients such as phycocyanin and beta-Carotene that possess antioxidant and anti-inflammatory properties. Phycocyanin can fight free-radicals as well as decrease nitrate production.[11]

Beta-Carotene is another antioxidant that protects against single oxygen-mediated lipid peroxidation and like phycocyanin is capable of inhibiting nitrate production. This protects the cells from the harmful effects of oxidation.

Studies have been done to test the effectiveness on spirulina on allergic rhinitis and in one such study done in Eskisehir Osmangazi University Medical Faculty in Turkey, spirulina was proven to be "clinically effective" in treating allergic rhinitis (inflamed sinuses from allergies) compared to placebo.[12]

Recent reports note the importance of spirulina for its immuno-modulatory, antifatigue and radio protective effects. Spirulina is commonly used in Asian cuisine. In America, spirulina is sold in health food stores as a powder or tablet. In Russia, it has been approved to treat symptoms of radiation sickness, because the carotenoids it contains absorb radiation.[13] Spirulina also is reported to slow neurological damage in aging animals, and also to lessen the damage caused by stroke.[14] Studies also show that spirulina can prevent the release of histamines, treating allergy symptoms.

The aqueous extract of spirulina was found to have a major impact on the immune system by increasing the phagocytic activity of macrophages (cells that devour bad bugs), stimulating the NK cells (immune cells that attack things like cancer). It also played a role in the activation and mobilization of T and B cells (immune cells that help fight infection) due to its stimulatory effects in the production of cytokines and antibodies.[15]

Spirulina reduces the severity and recovery of strokes. It also reverses age-related declines in memory and learning.[16]

According to the National Institutes of Health (NIH), many people promote Spirulina as a treatment for a range of metabolism and heart health issues, including weight loss, diabetes, and high cholesterol. People may also recommend it as an aid for various mental and emotional disorders, including anxiety, stress, depression, and attention deficit-hyperactivity disorder (ADHD).

NIH also reports Spirulina is said to help a range of eclectic health problems, including premenstrual symptoms and amyotrophic lateral sclerosis (Lou Gehrig's disease). In a combination mixed with zinc it may help the body clear arsenic in people whose drinking water has unusually high levels.

Spirulina is rich in nutrients, some of which aren't found in the average daily vitamin. According to the FDA, It contains significant amounts of calcium, niacin, potassium, magnesium, B vitamins, and iron. It also has essential amino acids (compounds that are the building blocks of proteins). In fact, protein makes up about 60 to 70 percent of its dry weight. This makes it especially beneficial for improving energy and repair.

Oligomeric proanthrocyanidin complexes (OPCs), are extremely potent antioxidant compounds and have been used successfully to improve a vast array of different health conditions. Studies show that OPCs provide many health benefits to the skin, including reducing the signs of aging.

Certain plants in nature contain these OPC compounds that produce very powerful and effective antioxidant capabilities. **Pine bark extract** contains beneficial amounts of these flavonoid compounds. **Pycnogenol** is a branded form of pine bark that is promoted for a number of uses including; skin healing and repair, rapid wound healing, improved circulation, joint pain, and in the prevention of cancer, to name a few. This is mainly attributed to its powerful antioxidant and anti-inflammatory properties. It is also used quite extensively in the antiaging community. In fact, a small 2012 study on postmenopausal women found that pycnogenol improved hydration and elasticity of skin. Study participants took pycnogenol as a supplement, and it was found to be most effective in women who started out with dry skin. The researchers concluded that pycnogenol may increase production of hyaluronic acid and collagen, which are both found in many popular antiaging products.[17]

A 2004 animal study also found that applying a gel containing pycnogenol sped up the wound-healing process. It also reduced the size of scars.[18] These findings may suggest it can be a useful supplement for individuals who have undergone surgery of any kind.

A 2017 review reported on the many benefits of using pycnogenol to reduce the effects of aging on skin.[19] Pycnogenol appears to reduce the creation of free radicals, which are molecules that cause oxidative damage especially to the skin. It also seems to help with cell regeneration and replication. Remember that the skin is a good representation of how healthy the body is on the inside. If these compounds are improving the skin, it's obvious it's adding a tremendous amount of benefit to the entire system as well.

In addition to its skin-healing properties, pycnogenol also shows promise for helping children manage ADHD symptoms. A 2006 study found that children who took a daily pycnogenol supplement for four weeks had significantly lower levels of hyperactivity. It also appeared to improve their attention span, visual motor skills, and concentration. The study participants' symptoms started to return a month after they stopped taking pycnogenol.[20] It seems the trend is to put kids on medications for their attention deficits instead of seeking more natural approaches. There are some pretty impressive studies, along with clinical results from my own practice and many of my colleagues included, that have demonstrated dramatic improvements, and in some cases complete normalization, in the kids who follow some of these more natural strategies.

The results of a 2013 animal study suggest that pycnogenol may help to reduce damage to nerve cells following a traumatic brain injury.[21] This is thought to be due to pycnogenol's ability to reduce oxidative stress and inflammation. What a great weapon to use in the fight against oxidation and inflammation. A 2015 review indicates that pycnogenol can be used to treat metabolic syndrome and related disorders such as obesity, diabetes, and high blood pressure.[22]

When oxidation is reduced in the body, the processes and conditions caused by them improve. It's just that simple.

There is another source in nature that also yields a high potency of OPCs and that is grape seed extract. **Grape seed extract (GSE) is** a dietary supplement made by removing, drying, and pulverizing the bitter tasting seeds. They are rich in antioxidants, including phenolic acids, anthrocyanins, flavonoids, and OPCs. GSE is one of the best-known sources of proanthocyanidins.[23] Due to its high antioxidant content, GSE can help protect against oxidative stress, tissue damage and inflammation.[24] When tissues are damaged and inflamed, GSE is the equivalent to applying a healing balm to the affected area bringing instant relief in many cases. The OPC content in the GSE travels through the bloodstream to block the harmful effects of oxidative stress while at the same time reducing inflammation. When people experience pain and inflammation, it's quite common to see an elevation in their blood pressure. A meta-analysis of 16 studies in 810 people with high blood pressures examined the effect of GSE on the condition. They found that 100-2,000 mg of GSE per day significantly reduced systolic blood pressure (the top number) by an average of 6.08 mmHg and diastolic (bottom number) by 2.8mmHg.[25] The most promising results came from lower doses of 100-800 mg daily for 8-17 weeks rather than a single dose of 800 mg or greater.[26]

There are countless people who suffer from pain and swelling in their legs and just learn to live with it. Many times they're given diuretics and pain pills that steal their energy and force them to live in a state of partial dehydration. An additional study in eight healthy young women assessed the effects of a single 400 mg dose of proanthrocyanidin from GSE followed by six hours of sitting. It was shown to reduce leg swelling and edema by 70 percent, compared to not taking GSE.[27]

In the same study, eight more healthy young women, who took a daily dose of 133 mg of the GSE for 14 days, experienced 40 percent less leg swelling after six hours of sitting.[28]

In another study. 61 healthy adults saw a 13.9 percent reduction in oxidized LDL after taking 400 mg of GSE.[29] Additionally, a study in 87 people undergoing heart surgery found that 400 mg of GSE given the day before surgery significantly reduced oxidative stress. Therefore, GSE likely protected against further heart damage.[30] Equipping the body with the tools it needs so it can protect itself from unwanted damage is an attainable goal if provided with the correct resources. OPCs are certainly a valid part of preventing these destructive processes in order to STOP THE PAIN.

There are obviously many different causes and processes that influence these types of disorders, but improving oxidation levels is a great first step in treating any condition.

N-acetyl cysteine is a sulfur containing amino acid that is also a very powerful antioxidant. This compound is extremely beneficial for people who have had chronic allergies, sinus problems, and even lung conditions due to its ability to break up mucous secretions. The most common use of NAC is for liver support in general, as an antioxidant, and detoxification due to the sulfur containing compound it possesses. Actually a 2010 study suggests NAC may be a better suited than resveratrol for using in patients with Hepatitis C virus and other chronic liver diseases.[31]

Some of its most promising uses are as a neuroprotectant. It is the precursor for the master antioxidant of the body, **glutathione**. This simply means when someone supplements with NAC the body converts it to glutathione as needed. Scientists are currently investigating it as a treatment for Parkinson's disease — a disorder that has been linked to glutathione deficiency.[32]

This deficiency is not restricted to Parkinson's, however. Subsequent studies have found this same type of glutathione deficiency is common in a number of other neurodegenerative conditions as well, including progressive supranuclear palsy, multiple system atrophy, and even Alzheimer's disease.[33]

In one small-scale clinical trial, 600 milligrams (mg) of intravenous glutathione was administered twice a day for 30 days, after which the patients were monitored for up to four months. All experienced significant improvement, with an average decline in disability of 42 percent.[34] NAC has been used to treat anything from sinus problems and severe neurodegenerative conditions, to preventing liver and kidney damage and improving immune function. Personally I believe that every person that has high levels of oxidation should be supplementing with this powerful nutrient.

Alpha lipoic acid (ALA) is an antioxidant that is often used clinically to help resensitize insulin receptors to decrease insulin resistance levels, which is extremely important for diabetics. It is well known as a potent and highly effective antioxidant. In several European countries, it used as an approved drug to treat diabetes-related complications, certain complications of alcoholism, and a variety of liver conditions.[35]

One of the major contributors of diabetes is the amount of oxidative stress and free radical damage associated with it. Lipoic acid has been shown to neutralize free radicals and reduce the oxidative stress to help prevent and reverse these damaging effects.[36] It also is capable of working in both fat soluble and water soluble mediums in the body, therefore making it easily absorbed and transported into organs, tissues, and systems like the liver, brain, nervous system.

Lipoic acid also enhances the effects of other antioxidants in the body. It promotes better absorption for vitamin C and E and actually regenerates them in the system. It also amplifies the powerful effects of other antioxidants such as glutathione and CoQ10. It works together with the B vitamins to help protect the mitochondria from oxidative stress during the conversion from food to energy so that energy production remains efficient. ALA is often combined with acetyl L carnitine to help promote the metabolism of fats and to assist the mitochondrial system in making energy more efficiently.

CoQ10 is a powerful antioxidant for the heart and other vital organs. It also plays a huge role in the production of energy by the mitochondria. Coenzyme Q10 is a member of the ubiquinone family of compounds. All animals, including humans, can synthesize ubiquinones, hence, coenzyme Q10 is not considered a vitamin.[37] In its reduced form ($CoQ10H2$), coenzyme Q10 is an effective fat-soluble antioxidant that protects cell membranes and lipoproteins from oxidation. The presence of a significant amount of $CoQ10H2$ in cell membranes, along with enzymes capable of reducing oxidized $CoQ10$ back to $CoQ10H2$, supports the idea that $CoQ10H2$ is an important cellular antioxidant.[38] $CoQ10H2$ has been found to inhibit lipid peroxidation when cell membranes and low-density lipoproteins (LDL) are exposed to oxidizing conditions. When LDL is oxidized, $CoQ10H2$ is the first antioxidant consumed. In isolated mitochondria, coenzyme Q10 can protect membrane proteins and mitochondrial DNA from the oxidative damage that accompanies lipid peroxidation.[39]

Lysosomes are organelles that are working components within cells that are specialized for the digestion of cellular debris (waste). They (lysosomes) contain digestive enzymes that function best at a specific pH range (acidic). The membranes that separate those digestive enzymes from the rest of the cell contain relatively high concentrations of coenzyme Q10. Research suggests that coenzyme Q10 plays an important role in the transport of protons across lysosomal membranes to maintain the optimal pH.[40] A simpler way to understand this is; CoQ10 plays an important part in managing and maintaining the janitorial crew of the body that cleans up the mess that's made during normal daily operation of the cells. This allows the body to make energy much more efficiently. This is one of the most important things to correct when trying to recover from chronic pain syndromes, sickness, and/or addictions. The rate of repair cannot exceed the rate of damage if the body doesn't have enough energy to perform the functions needed to heal itself. CoQ10 is a vital part of restoring this process.

According to the free radical and mitochondrial theories of aging, oxidative damage of cell structures by reactive oxygen species (ROS) plays an important role in the functional declines that accompany aging.[41] ROS are generated by mitochondria as a by-product of ATP (energy) production. If not neutralized by antioxidants, ROS may damage mitochondria over time, causing them to function less efficiently and to generate more damaging ROS in a self-perpetuating cycle. Coenzyme Q10 plays an important role in mitochondrial ATP synthesis and functions as an antioxidant in mitochondrial membranes to block this damaging cycle. One of the hallmarks of aging is a decline in energy metabolism in many tissues, especially liver, heart, and skeletal muscle. This natural progression is one of the major reasons we start to "feel old." Tissue concentrations of coenzyme Q10 have been found to decline with age, thereby accompanying age-related declines in energy metabolism.[42] Without proper levels of CoQ10, the body can't keep up the pace of a youthful metabolism. However, in a small randomized controlled trial, elderly individuals (>70 years) who received a combination of selenium (100 mg/day) and coenzyme Q10 (200 mg/day) for four years reported an improvement in vitality, physical performance, and quality of life.[43] It's quite obvious from the research that CoQ10 has the potential to block damaging effects from oxidation, protect the mitochondria by helping to maintain them and keep them working efficiently, and helps improve the function and vitality that declines during the aging process. Maybe you can't add years to your life, but supplementing with antioxidants like CoQ10 and selenium, you can add life to your years.

Lutein is the antioxidant that has been shown to stop macular degeneration. It is believed that when lutein, zeaxanthin and me-so-zeaxanthin are combined in the macula, they work together to block blue light from reaching the underlying structures in the retina, thereby reducing the risk of light-induced oxidative damage that could lead to macular degeneration (AMD). The carotenoid **lutein** has long been studied for its vision-protective properties. It has been shown to reduce the risk of two of the leading causes of blindness: age-related macular degeneration and cataracts.[44]

A recent study has revealed that we've only scratched the surface of lutein's health-promoting benefits. In a first-of-its-kind analysis, lutein has been associated with a reduced risk for **cardio metabolic diseases**.

A large meta-analysis involving **71 published papers** and representing more than **387,000 individuals** showed that people with higher lutein intake, or higher blood concentrations of lutein, have a reduced risk of coronary heart disease, stroke, and metabolic syndrome.[45]

The reason lutein provides such wide-reaching effects is because of its ability to protect tissues from oxidative stress and inflammation—two factors that play a major role in cardiovascular and metabolic diseases.

This study will likely change the way we think of lutein, broadening its appeal to everyone who wants to optimally protect their blood vessels, heart, and brain against the ravages of oxidative stress and chronic inflammation.

Ginkgo biloba is a very powerful plant, and it is especially good for stopping brain inflammation. It helps promote good circulation (helps blood profuse) to the brain, so you get more nutrients there. It actually crosses the blood-brain barrier. Most nutraceuticals do not. According to the University of Maryland Medical Center (UMM), "Ginkgo is widely used in Europe for treating dementia." Doctors started to use it because they thought it improved blood flow to the brain, but more recent studies indicate that it may protect nerve cells from damage in Alzheimer's as well.

Standardized extracts of Ginkgo biloba leaves possess antioxidant properties that act as a free radical scavenger. It was originated by Dr. Willmar Schwabe Pharmaceuticals (Dr. Willmar Schwabe group) and has been available in Europe as a herbal extract since the early 1990s.[46] In Norway products of Ginkgo leaf have actually been approved by the Norwegian Medicines Agency to improve blood circulation.[47]

Ginkgo biloba can be very useful for people who suffer with chronic pain and soreness as it improves the circulation providing fresh oxygenated blood to the painful areas reducing stiffness, soreness, and pain.

Citrus Bioflavonoids

Citrus bioflavonoids are compounds that exist in fruits and vegetables that are often found coupled together vitamin C within nature. Citrus bioflavonoids help tonify ligaments. They also help tighten up tissues.

Bioflavonoids have antioxidant properties thought to be particularly beneficial for capillary strength. Bioflavonoids from citrus fruits are believed to work with vitamin C to promote immune system health.[48] Compounds commonly featured in citrus bioflavonoid supplements include hesperidin, rutin, naringin, and quercetin. These phytonutrients are thought to be vital for proper absorption of Vitamin C.[49] Citrus Bioflavonoids are typically used in health supplements to support the immune system.[50] Bioflavonoids are used as an aid to enhance the action of vitamin C, to support blood circulation, as antioxidants, and to treat allergies, viruses, or arthritis and other inflammatory conditions.[51] A 1955 study by Dr. Biskind looked at 69 cases of acute respiratory infections that were treated with a whole water soluble citrus bioflavonoid complex. The disorders included the common cold, acute follicular tonsillitis, and influenza. Within 8 to 48 hours all but three cases saw a significant decline in infection. Dr. Biskind credited this rapid recovery to improved capillary permeability and the enhanced vitamin C bioavailability.[52] In 1962, Dr. Robert Cragin used lemon-orange derived bioflavonoids on different groups of athletes in a double-blind study. It was found that the athletes taking bioflavonoids experienced less muscle and joint injuries than the control group. These athletes also recovered quicker from similar injuries than the group of athletes not taking the bioflavonoids. The addition of vitamin C to the bioflavonoids (as seen in citrus fruits) appeared to enhance these effects.[53]

Studies have shown benefits of the citrus bioflavonoids on capillary permeability and blood flow. This is likely due to the powerful anti-inflammatory effects of these phytonutrients. This is especially important for oxygenating tissues and maintaining normal blood pressure. They also reduce swelling, venous backup, and edema. This process frequently improves respiration in the lungs.[54] Based on the research alone one can see how beneficial these compounds can be for anyone who has degenerative and/or debilitating and even chronic pain syndromes.

You can find bioflavonoids in the pulp and white core that runs through the center of citrus fruits, green peppers, lemons, limes, oranges, cherries, and grapes. Quercetin is a highly concentrated form of bioflavonoids found in broccoli, citrus fruits, and red and yellow onions. Flavonoids, which include resveratrol, proanthocyanidin, quercetin and catechin, may be at least partly responsible for the health benefits of a diet rich in fruits and vegetables.

Over the past thirty years I have personally witnessed countless numbers of people who have recovered from devastating chronic degenerative and even acute aggressive conditions from administering combined antioxidant therapies. I have had many discussions with fellow practitioners who have shared the same results. Whether taken orally or administered by injection or IV, antioxidants can have a profound effect on your health.

Detecting and correcting the problems in the antioxidant system is not only essential, but also paramount in recovering from painful, degenerative, and destructive conditions in the body. It's also of equal importance in order to stay healthy once you obtain a healthy status.

In my opinion, oxidation and inflammation are two of the most significant mechanisms for causing pain, degeneration, and disease. They are constantly working against us, and if we want to preserve health, we should do whatever it takes to keep them under control. Everyone should be doing something to control them. The question is. "Where do you start?" I have learned that if you want to change something, you have to have a strategy. So a good start at this point would be to do the pain stoppers.

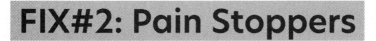

FIX#2: Pain Stoppers

- Take out the bad fats, put in the good ones.

- Start taking some enzymes to help digest the food.

- Add into the diet some or all of the nutrient compounds discussed that apply to your particular needs.

- Have your vitamin D levels evaluated to see if your vitamin D3 blood values are low or if the receptors are resistant and restore any imbalances that may exist.

- Add digestive enzymes and the compounds discussed that help to digest and assimilate the fats.

- Add the nutrients and compounds discussed that help repair and restore the microbiome and assist with proper bowel function.

- Include live fresh foods, preferably raw, every day with meals.

- Follow this regimen for a few weeks.

- Do the gallbladder flush and follow with the coffee enema.

- After completing that, add some antioxidants to the diet, such as the ones you just read about and remove the destructive things from your life that provoke this vicious cycle. It's pretty simple. Follow the instructions in the book, stay consistent, and start your journey on the road to recovery.

STOP THE PAIN: The Six to Fix

1. Vitamin E slows down the progression of osteoarthritis XI LI, ZHONGLI DONG, [...], and YUAN ZHANG Exp Ther Med 2016 Jul ;12(1) :18-22.

2. Ellagitannins from Raspberry (Rubus idaeus L.) Fruit as Natural Inhibitors of Geotrichum candidum; Elz bieta Klewicka , Michał Sójka , Robert Klewicki, Krzysztof Kołodziejczyk , Lidia Lipinska and Adriana Nowak, Academic Editor: Isabel C. F. R. Ferreira. Received: 30 May 2016; Accepted: 8 July 2016; Published: 13 July 2016.

3. Ellagitannins Renewed the Concept of Tannins; Takuo Okuda,* a Takashi Yoshida,b Tsutomu Hatanoc and Hideyuki Itoca Emeritus Professor, Okayama University, Okayama 700-8530, Japan; bCollege of Pharmaceutical Sciences, Matsuyama University, Bunkyo-cho, Matsuyama, Ehime 790-8578, Japan; cDepartment of Pharmacognosy, Okayama University Graduate School of Medicine, Dentistry and Pharmaceutical Sciences, Tsushima, Okayama 700-8530.

4. Haslam, 1989, Okuda, 1995, 1999a, 2005, Okuda et. al., 1990, 1991, 1992a, 1993a, 1995, 2000, Quideau and Feldman, 1996).

5. Miyamoto et. al., 1997.

6. Inoue et. al., 1994, Sakagami et al., 1995, 1999.

7. Miyamoto et. al., 1993, see Chapter 6.

8. National Nutrient Database for Standard Reference 1 Release April, 2018.

9. Ergogenic and antioxidant effects of spirulina supplementation in humans. Kalafati M1, Jamurtas AZ, Nikolaidis MG, Paschalis V, Theodorou AA, Sakellariou GK, Koutedakis Y, Kouretas D.Med Sci Sports Exerc. 2010 Jan; 42(1):142-51. doi: 10.1249/MSS.0b013e3181ac7a45.

10. Role of Spirulina in the Control of Glycemia and Lipidemia in Type 2 Diabetes Mellitus. Parikh P1, Mani U, Iyer U. J Med Food. 2001 Winter;4(4):193-199.

11. Hypolipidemic, Antioxidant and anti-inflammatory activities of Microalgae Spirulina Cardiovascular Ther. 2010 Aug.;28(4):e33-e45.

12. The effects of spirulina on allergic rhinitis. Cingi C1, Conk-Dalay M, Cakli H, Bal C. Eur Arch Otorhinolaryngol. 2008 Oct;265(10):1219-23. doi: 10.1007/s00405-008-0642-8. Epub 2008 Mar 15.

13. Cifferi O. Spirulina as a micro organism. Microbiol Rev. 1983;47(4): 551-578.

14. Wang Y, Chen-Fu C, Chou J, et al. Dietary supplementation with blueberries, spinach, or spirulina reduces ischemic brain damage. Experiment Neurol. 2005;193(1):75–84.

15. Schwartz J, Shklar G. Regression of experimental hamster cancer by beta carotene and algae extracts. J Oral Maxillofac Surg. 1987 Jun;45(6): 510-515.

16. Nemoto-Kawamura C, Hirahashi T, Nagai T, Yamada H, Katoh T, Hayashi O. Phycocyanin enhances secretary IgA antibody response and suppresses allergic IgE antibody response in mice immunized with antigen-entrapped biodegradable microparticles. J Nutr Sci Vitaminol (Tokyo). 2004;50(2):129–136 Cingi C, Conk-Dalay M, Cakli H, Bal C. The effects of Spirulina on allergic rhinitis. Err Arch Oto-Rhino-Larynol 2008;265(10) 1219-1223.

17. Pycnogenol effects on Skin Elasticity and Hydration Coincide with increased Gene Expressions of Collagen Type 1 and Hyaluronic Acid Synthase in Women.

18. Pycnogenol accelerates wound healing and reduces scar formation First published:03 August 2004, available at http://doi.org/10.1002/par.1477 cited by: 29.

19. Pycnogenol: A Miracle Component in Reducing Aging and Skin Disorders Chowdhury WK,Arne S,Debnath S,Alija T,Khan A, et. al.(2017). J Clin Exp Dermatol Res 8:395.doi10.4172/2155-9554.1000395.

20. Treatment of ADHD with French maritime pine bark extract, Pycnogenol Jana Trebaticka, Sona Kopasova, Zuzuna Hradecna, Kamil Cinovsky, Jan Suba, Jana Muchová, Ingrid Zitnanova, Iveta Waczulikova, Peter Rohdewald, Zdenka Durackova Europe on Child & Adolescent Psychology Sept 2006,volume 15,issue 6, pp 329-335.

21. Neuroprotective effect of Pycnogenol following traumatic brain injury Steven W. Schiff, Mubeen A. Ansari, Kelly N Roberts available at http://doi.org/10.1016/j.expneurol.2012.09.019.

22. Pycnogenol in Metabolic Syndrome and Related Disorders Or P. Gulati 01 May 2015 available at https://doi.org/10.1002/PTL.5341 cited by:9.

23. Proanthocyanidin-rich grape seed extract reduces leg swelling in healthy women during prolonged sitting. Sano A1, Tokutake S, Seo A..J Sci Food Agric 2013 Feb;93(3):457-62. doi: 10.1002/jsfa.5773. Epub 2012 Jul 2 Atherosclerosis:processes, Indicators, Risk factors, and New Hopes Int J prev med. 2014 Aug;5(8):927-946.

24. Grape seed and skin extract reduces pancreas lipotoxicity, oxidative stress, and inflammation in high fat diet fed rats.

25. Aloui F1, Charradi K2, Hichami A3, Subramaniam S3, Khan NA3, Limam F4, Aouani E1. .Biomed Pharmacother. 2016 Dec;84:2020-2028. doi: 10.1016/j.biopha.2016.11.017. Epub 2016 Nov 12.

26. Protective effects of grape seed and skin extract against high-fat-diet-induced lipotoxicity in rat lung. El Ayed M1, Kadri S2, Smine S2,3, Elkahoui S2, Limam F2, Aouani E2.Lipids Health Dis. 2017 Sep 13;16(1):174. doi: 10.1186/s12944-017-0561-z.

27. Protective effect of grape seed and skin extract against high-fat diet-induced liver steatosis and zinc depletion in rat. Charradi K1, Elkahoui S, Karkouch I, Limam F, Ben Hassine F, El May MV, Aouani E. Dig Dis Sci. 2014 Aug;59(8):1768-78. doi: 10.1007/s10620-014-3128-0. Epub 2014 Apr 6.

28. Beneficial effects of grape seed extract on malondialdehyde-modified LDL. Sano A1, Uchida R, Saito M, Shioya N, Komori Y, Tho Y, Hashizume N. J Nutr Sci Vitaminol (Tokyo). 2007 Apr;53(2):174-82.

29. Effect of a standardized grape seed extract on low-density lipoprotein susceptibility to oxidation in heavy smokers. Vigna GB1, Costantini F, Aldini G, Carini M, Catapano A, Schena F, Tangerini A, Zanca R, Bombardelli E, Morazzoni P, Mezzetti A, Fellin R, Maffei Facino R. Metabolism. 2003 Oct;52(10):1250-7.

30. Grape seed proanthocyanidins prevent plasma postprandial oxidative stress in humans. Natella F1, Belelli F, Gentili V, Ursini F, Scaccini C. J Agric Food Chem. 2002 Dec 18;50(26):7720-5.

31. Comparative effect of grape seed extract (Vitis vinifera) and ascorbic acid in oxidative stress induced by on-pump coronary artery bypass surgery. Safaei N1, Babaei H2, Azarfarin R3, Jodati AR1, Yaghoubi A3, Sheikhalizadeh MA1.Ann Card Anaesth. 2017 Jan-Mar;20(1):45-51. doi: 10.4103/0971-9784.197834.

32. World Journal of Gastroenterology : WJG Baishideng Publishing Group Inc Hepatoprotective effects of antioxidants in chronic hepatitis C Ricardo Moreno-Otero and María Trapero-Marugán Neuroscience letters 1982 Dec 13;33(3):305-10.

33. Movement disorders 2003 Sep ;18(9);969-76.

34. Prof neuropsychoparmacol Biol Psychiatry 1996 Oct;20(7):1159-70.

35. http://www.pdrhealth.com/drug_info/nmdrugprofiles/nutsupdrugs/alp_0159.shtml. Accessed July 16, 2007 Da Ros R,Ceriello A. Molecular targets of diabetic vascular complications and potential new drugs.Curr Drug Targets. 2005 Jun;6(4):503-9.

36. Ceriello A. New insights on oxidative stress and diabetic complications may lead to "causal" antioxidant therapy. Diabetes Care . 2003 May;26(5):1589-96.

37. Acosta MJ, Vazquez Fonseca L, Desbats MA, et al. Coenzyme Q biosynthesis in health and disease. Biochim Biophys Acta. 2016;1857(8):1079-1085. (PubMed).

38. Navas P, Villalba JM, de Cabo R. The importance of plasma membrane coenzyme Q in aging and stress responses. Mitochondrion. 2007;7 Suppl:S34-40. (PubMed).

39. Ernster L, Dallner G. Biochemical, physiological and medical aspects of ubiquinone function. Biochim Biophys Acta. 1995;1271(1):195-204. (PubMed).

40. Crane FL. Biochemical functions of coenzyme Q10. J Am Coll Nutr. 2001;20(6):591-598. (PubMed) Nohl H, Gille L. The role of coenzyme Q in lysosomes. In: Kagan VEQ, P. J., ed. Coenzyme Q: Molecular Mechanisms in Health and Disease. Boca Raton: CRC Press; 2001:99-106.

41. Beckman KB, Ames BN. Mitochondrial aging: open questions. Ann N Y Acad Sci. 1998;854:118-127. (PubMed).

42. Kalén A, Appelkvist EL, Dallner G. Age-related changes in the lipid compositions of rat and human tissues. Lipids. 1989;24(7):579-584. (PubMed).

43. Johansson P, Dahlstrom O, Dahlstrom U, Alehagen U. Improved health-related quality of life, and more days out of hospital with supplementation with selenium and coenzyme Q10 combined. Results from a double-blind, placebo-controlled prospective study. J Nutr Health Aging. 2015;19(9):870-877. (PubMed).

44. Scripsema NK, Hu DN, Rosen RB. Lutein, zeaxanthin, and meso-zeaxanthin in the clinical management of eye disease. *J Ophthalmol.* 2015;2015:865179.

Abdel-Aal el SM, Akhtar H, Zaheer K, et. al. Dietary sources of lutein and zeaxanthin carotenoids and their role in eye health. *Nutrients.* 2013;5(4):1169-85.

45. Leermakers ET, Darweesh SK, Baena CP, et al. The effects of lutein on cardiometabolic health across the life course: a systematic review and meta-analysis. *Am J Clin Nutr.* 2016;103(2):481-94. *Kijlstra* A, Tian Y, Kelly ER, et al. Lutein: more than just a filter for blue light. *Prog Retin Eye Res.* 2012;31(4):303-15. Sujak A, Gabrielska J, Grudzinski W, et. al. Lutein and zeaxanthin as protectors of lipid membranes against oxidative damage: the structural aspects. *Arch Biochem Biophys.* 1999;371(2):301-7.

46. Drugs R D. 2003;4(3):188-93. EGb 761: ginkgo biloba extract, Ginkor. [No authors listed]Tidsskr Nor Laegeforen. 2012 Apr 30;132(8):956-9. doi: 10.4045/tidsskr.11.0780. [Ginkgo biloba--effect, adverse events and drug interaction].(pub med) [Article in Norwegian] Roland PD1, Nergård CS.

47. Tidsskr Nor Laegeforen. 2012 Apr 30;132(8):956-9. doi: 10.4045/tidsskr.11.0780.[Ginkgo biloba--effect, adverse events and drug interaction].(pub med) [Article in Norwegian]Roland PD1, Nergård CS.

48. Antioxidant Capacity, Anticancer Ability and Flavonoids Composition of 35 Citrus (Citrus reticulata Blanco) Varieties. Wang Y, Qian J, Cao J, Wang D, Liu C, Yang R, Li X, Sun C. Molecules. 2017 Jul 5;22(7). pii: E1114. doi: 10.3390/molecules22071114.

49. Anti-Inflammatory and Neuroprotective Constituents from the Peels of Citrus grandis. Kuo PC, Liao YR, Hung HY, Chuang CW, Hwang TL, Huang SC, Shiao YJ, Kuo DH, Wu TS. Molecules. 2017 Jun 9;22(6). pii: E967. doi: 10.3390/molecules22060967.

50. Bioavailable Citrus sinensis Extract: Polyphenolic Composition and Biological Activity. Pepe G, Pagano F, Adesso S, Sommella E, Ostacolo C, Manfra M, Chieppa M, Sala M, Russo M, Marzocco S, Campiglia P. Molecules. 2017 Apr 15;22(4). pii: E623. doi: 10.3390/molecules22040623.

51. C-Glycosyltransferases catalyzing the formation of di-C-glucosyl flavonoids in citrus plants. Ito T, Fujimoto S, Suito F, Shimosaka M, Taguchi G. Plant J. 2017 Jul;91(2):187-198. doi: 10.1111/tpj.13555. Epub 2017 Jun 5.

52. The Citrus Flavanone Naringenin Produces Cardioprotective Effects in Hearts from 1 Year Old Rat, through Activation of mitoBK Channels. Testai L, Da Pozzo E, Piano I, Pistelli L, Gargini C, Breschi MC, Braca A, Martini C, Martelli A, Calderone V. Front Pharmacol. 2017 Feb 27;8:71. doi: 10.3389/fphar.2017.00071. eCollection 2017.

53. The effects of flavanone-rich citrus juice on cognitive function and cerebral blood flow: an acute, randomised, placebo-controlled cross-over trial in healthy, young adults. Lamport DJ, Pal D, Macready AL, Barbosa-Boucas S, Fletcher JM, Williams CM, Spencer JP, Butler LT. Br J Nutr. 2016 Dec;116(12):2160-2168. doi: 10.1017/S000711451600430X. Epub 2017 Jan 16.

54. Bioactive compounds in foods: their role in the prevention of cardiovascular disease and cancer. Kris-Etherton PM, Hecker KD, Bonanome A, Coval SM, Binkoski AE, Hilpert KF, Griel AE, Etherton TD. Am J Med. 2002 Dec 30;113 Suppl 9B:71S-88S. Review.

IMMUNE RESPONSE

Immune Responses

Eliminate the "Big Three" from Diet

The grandest portals of entry to the inside of the body are the nose and mouth. The mouth is primarily composed of lips for sealing the entrance, teeth for support and chewing, and a tongue for facilitation of multiple tasks from forming sounds to positioning and moving food around for chewing. I prefer to call the nose and mouth "The Gateways to Health."

The Gateways to Health

The oxygen-rich air and the foods and beverages we consume that contain the life-sustaining nutrients we require to stay alive, as well as healthy, pass through these gates on their way to be delivered to the body. Every entry into the body must have some sort of detection-protection surveillance system or invading substances that were not designed to be there might find their way to the inside. The primary portal entryways to the human body are the mouth, nose, and skin. All three of these portals allow substances to pass through their entryways, which are lined with sensitive tissue cells (**epithelial tissue**), allowing them to have access in and out of the body. In the epithelial linings of each of these entryways, there are detective-protective surveillance systems that sound the alarm when invaders try to pass through. These systems are composed of different cells (**dendritic cells**) and lymphatic tissue that communicate with the body's immune system once an invader has been detected. Upon detection of an intruder, these cells release chemical proteins called cytokines that travel to the immune system to sound the alarm.

The body responds by releasing a barrage of immune cells that rapidly travel through the body to greet the intruder. Once encountered, the invading substance is coded, marked, and either destroyed, stored, or altered to be a safe substance. The immune system keeps record of the intruder and forms immunity to it for future reference.

In the mouth and digestive tract, the immune detection and protection surveillance system is referred to as the **Gut Associated Lymphatic Tissue (G.A.L.T)**. This same system in the nasal passages and pulmonary system is called the **Nasal Associated Lymphatic Tissue (N.A.L.T)**. In the skin this system is called the **Skin Associated Lymphatic Tissue (S.A.L.T)**. Like scanners at the airport, they attempt to prevent harmful passengers from getting on board.

If a foreign substance tries to pass through and is recognized as unfriendly to the body, these systems sound the alarm and respond by releasing chemical messengers called "cytokines." Cytokines are composed of protein and their primary purpose is to signal cells to affect other cells. Some cytokines have constructive effects and some have destructive effects, depending upon which system signals which type.

The Good, the Bad, and the Ugly

When one of the gateways signal these cytokine messengers to provoke an immune response, the immune system releases the appropriate army of cells to command an attack on the unfriendly intruder. Depending upon the severity of the contamination, the immune
response can often be quite severe. Here is a hypothetical situation
of how immune responses can cause the body to label things, such
as food, that are intended to provide nourishment instead get labeled as "bad guys." This in turn causes the body to set up a defense
mechanism against them. The foods that get labeled are treated as
foreign invaders and cause what medical science refers to as "food
sensitivities." Once these reactions are generated in the body, they
can lead to a variety of symptoms and, if not managed properly, can
progress into sickness and disease.

Let us pretend for a moment that you are on the inside of your gut
and a few contaminated chunks of potato have been ingested. The
body immediately unleashes an attack as the G.A.L.T. sounds the
alarm. Now a war is raging between your immune system and potentially harmful bacteria such as E. coli that the potato was contaminated with.

Things are getting pretty hectic as the battle rages on. The good
immune cells are trying to mark all of the bad guys so that the army
that has been deployed by the immune system can destroy them,
but during the process, somehow, some of the chunks of potato
get marked as well. The body then codes those potato chunks as
unfriendly. Let us also suppose that during this same process, that
even some of the gut tissue cells got marked as well. The body codes
those cells as unfriendly. Fast forward three months later. The battle
in the gut has been long forgotten and you are feeling great. You
decide you are hungry and you go out for a bowl of soup. Not even

aware of the potential consequence you are facing, you order a bowl of potato soup with crackers. The soup enters through the gateway to health and passes into the gut. The G.A.L.T. immediately releases a barrage of cytokine messengers to the immune system as it has detected the potato and remembers that it was coded as unfriendly a few months prior. The next thing you know, the immune system is deploying an army of cells to attack the unfriendly intruder and "BOOM," you are right back where you were a few months prior. You just went from feeling great to experiencing symptoms in your body as if you were sick. Automatically you assume that the cause must just be from some virus that is going around. A few days later you recover, but you never realize that it was a food sensitivity caused by the potato that initiated the response. To make matters worse, when the potato was under attack from eating the soup, the body also coded some of the cracker molecules causing them to be coded as unfriendly. It was bad enough that you were sensitive to potatoes, but now you are sensitive to wheat as well. Over time as these foods are ingested, your body continues to code other foods as unfriendly and the food sensitivity list grows longer.

Through this entire scenario the gut cells that were coded as un-friendly continue to be re-attacked each time one of the coded foods are ingested. Chronically, over time the bowel begins to get irritated because of the damage from these recurrent attacks. You go to the doctor and he diagnoses you with **irritable bowel syndrome**. Didn't you kind of already know your bowel was irritable before you paid him to tell you that? Never-the-less, you accept your new diagnosis and continue in the same destructive eating habits and the damage continues. If this sensitivity problem remains undetect-ed, it can cause massive amounts of damage to the gut linings and even progress into disorders such as ulcerative colitis (bleeding and severe inflammation of the colon) and possibly even Crohn's disease (parts of the gastrointestinal tract become diseased due to chronic inflammation). Most people have a variety of symptoms because the gut is tied to so many other body functions.

Continuing on with this saga, matters get even more complicated. A couple of months later, you are at the grocery store and you are attempting to shop in a healthy manner. You are picking out a variety of vegetables. You see the potatoes and you put a few in your bag. On the way home from the grocery store, your eyes are feeling a bit tired and you rub them. You get home and start to put away the groceries and you notice a rash on your arm. The next thing you know your eyes are itching. What is wrong? You were feeling great, what happened? The detective protective system in the gut (G.A.L.T.) is also in the skin (S.A.L.T.). The same type cells release cytokine messengers and cause another immune response and now the symptoms have returned and the sensitivity cycles complete themselves once again.

Let us say that you are in a store and walk out to go to your car and as you come out of the door, there is a huge cloud of cigarette smoke lingering from the last person who was smoking. You walk through it and, immediately, you start to fan the offensive smell away from your nostrils, but the fact is you breathed a good bit of it in before you could get to fresh air. A few minutes later, you start to get the same reaction as when you were eating the potato. How is this possible? The nasal passages also have the same detective protective surveillance system (N.A.L.T.) as the gut. Tobacco is in the nightshade family. A potato is also in the **nightshade family**. Therefore, the N.A.L.T. detected the tobacco and coded it the same as the potato and released a cytokine response, which, in turn, provoked an immediate response from the immune system causing a sensitivity reaction and another internal war.

It's quite common to see these same sensitivities be reactivated and initiated from different sources. For example, you may have a sensitivity to corn and have been diligent to keep it out of the diet for several weeks. You haven't had any reactions and as a result you've been symptom-free. Let's say you breathe some corn dust when you sweep the floor of the barn. BOOM! You get a reaction and your symptoms flare back up again. What just happened? Do you remember the N.A.L.T. in the lining of the sinuses? It has the same security system as the G.A.L.T. does in your gut. Once it detected the corn dust, it labeled it as a repeat offender and sent a message to the immune system to sound the alarm. The corn dust has just been targeted for engagement. Once the immune activation is initiated, you start to swell, the symptoms return, and the whole process repeats itself.

Here is another wrench to throw into the gears. There is a 20-24 hour or longer gut transient time that can cause a delayed sensitivity. Sometimes you can eat a food and think you are fine, and you will not feel the reaction for a day or two, sometimes up to three days later. This really makes it challenging because it's hard to pinpoint which food caused the reaction.

Imagine living your life each and every day with these types of sensitivity reactions reoccurring continually. Is it a little easier to understand why so many people have so many unexplained symptoms? Can you see why there are so many misdiagnoses? I would dare to say that almost every person deals with sensitivities to some degree. The sensitivities cause inflammation in the system. When the body stays inflamed chronically, it can also produce pain and discomfort in the joints and muscles, which can progress into headaches, migraines, fibromyalgia, neck and back pain, and all sorts of pain and fatigue syndromes. How many times have you been feeling great with no aches or pains, plenty of energy, and a fresh, clear thought process? You may have even been bragging to people about how good you feel. You stop and get something to eat and a few minutes later, everything changes. Right after eating that meal you start to get tired, you lose all of your energy, and a few minutes later they can't even scrape you off of the couch. It is not rocket science! Something has to be in the food that is dramatically affecting you, but isn't it amazing how fast things can change once you put the wrong thing in the body?

> ❝When you put the right things in and you take the wrong things out, your body can often rapidly heal itself.❞

When you put the right things in and you take the wrong things out, your body can often rapidly heal itself. If the lining in the gut becomes damaged from being exposed to the wrong things, there is a way to repair it. There is an amino acid called **L-glutamine** which is what the body utilizes to heal and repair the epithelial lining of the gut. It requires a pretty high dose to repair a really sensitive gut. The current clinical research recommends doses as high as 25-30 grams daily. This would be considered a **clinical dose**. I personally have recommended this dose for many of my patients and they have experienced no ill effects. This dose should be maintained for an average of about three to six months until the gut has repaired itself. **Butyrate** is another compound that assists the gut in the healing process. It is a medium chain fatty acid that is used by the body to heal the linings in the colon. This combination seems to be quite effective for repairing damaged gut linings. Athletes quite commonly take higher doses of branch chain amino acids after strenuous exercise as they are what the body utilizes to heal and repair skeletal muscles. This is the same principle, using L-glutamine to target healing and repair of the gut. People with less damaged linings can certainly receive benefit from using lower dosages. The higher doses have been shown to be safe and effective and are used quite commonly in clinical settings. Anyone suffering with chronic gut inflammation, sinus and allergy problems, thyroid problems, and/or chronic digestive issues, should definitely consider L-glutamine to be included as a part of the treatment regimen.

DEFEAT THE WHEAT

One of the food sensitivities that has gained significant notoriety in recent years is wheat. Wheat has a protein component called gluten. Over the last several years more and more companies are buying wheat that has been genetically modified, which is altered from its original state and content. The **G.M.O. (Genetically Modified Organism)** wheat has an increase in gluten content compared to natural, unaltered wheat. This increased amount of gluten content is believed to cause significant antigen responses leading to severe sensitivity reactions in a large portion of our population.

Gluten is not limited to wheat but, in fact, exists in most grains and grain products. When someone has formed sensitivity to gluten and they consume most any grain, they are likely to experience a sensitivity reaction called a cross-reactivity reaction.

Most all of these sensitivity reactions can be detected by a simple blood test called an IgA/IgG food sensitivity panel, and if necessary, a cross-reactivity panel can be ordered as well. Typically, when a 96-food panel is done, it provides a pretty good understanding of which foods and which types of foods need to be eliminated from the diet initially. When sensitivities are present, especially the ones that score the most sensitive on the test, they need to be removed so the membranes have a chance to recover. It is kind of like when you get a sunburn on your skin. Normally, you can tolerate all kinds of things rubbing against your skin and you barely feel them. When you have a sunburn, however, even the slightest pressure from things rubbing against the skin can cause significant irritation. So it is with your gut or sinuses once they become inflamed. They become more sensitive. After a period of time of removing these irritating substances from the gut, it then has time to heal and the inflammation subsides. After the inflammation reduces or is resolved, the gut lining is far less sensitive and the symptoms reduce or resolve as well.

For nearly thirty years I have watched patients who follow the recommendations given and the results have been astonishing. Gut, bowel, sinus, skin problems, migraines, even pain and inflammation sometimes completely resolve and the other symptoms they were having completely go away as well. Many of those patients that were having symptoms never could have imagined the cause of those problems could be related to sensitivity reactions. Sometimes they would even get upset because they had been to many health professionals and had tried so many treatments and were no better or even worse after the treatments. Often they had a hard time believing that all of their complex issues could be coming from something as simple as a sensitivity reaction.

Novak Djokovic, the number one ranked professional tennis player in the world for several years in a row, removed gluten from his diet and, as a result, he was able to move up quickly to the number one spot when previously he had been stuck in the lower rankings. In his book, *Serve to Win*, he openly admitted that removing the gluten and dealing with that sensitivity reaction was one of the single most beneficial factors that propelled him to the top of one of the most competitive sports in the world. He claims that by removing the gluten products from his diet that his allergies, asthma, and

chronic fatigue all disappeared. If something that seems so insignif-
icant can create a world champion, just think of what it could do for
the lifestyle of the average person. Can you imagine having more
energy, more endurance, more stamina, no pain, and no symptoms?
The purpose of this book is to inform you of processes that could be
occurring in your body that you can detect and correct so you can
be restored to health and STOP THE PAIN!

Perhaps you are one of those individuals who is having sensitivity
reactions and had no idea they even existed until now. Maybe you
knew about them but you never thought that they could have such a
dramatic impact on your body's function and performance. Whatever the case, now that you know, you can start down the path to
health, healing, and recovery.

There are many things that can cause inflammation in the body.
Sensitivity reactions, infection, deficiencies, allergies, toxicity, and
even biomechanical disturbances, to name a few, can all provoke
inflammatory responses in the body. Food sensitivities are one of
the most common causes of chronic inflammation, but most of
the time, there are other concomitant processes occurring simultaneously that contribute to the inflammatory cascade. People are
constantly bombarded with all sorts of interactions that provoke
inflammatory responses. How many times have you rubbed your
eyes and a few minutes later they begin to itch? Perhaps another
instance, you jar your body by stepping off of a curb while crossing
the street, and a little while later, you start to experience back pain.
How about the times when you smell strong odors such as perfume,
chemical sprays, or even smoke, and a few minutes later you start to
develop a headache? All of these occurrences lead to inflammatory
responses that stimulate pain receptors in your nervous system and
cause a variety of pain syndromes as a result. Every day people are
influenced by these types of reactions and have no idea what caus-

es them and, for the most part, attempt to treat the symptoms, not the cause of their problems, in order to obtain relief. After years of treating symptoms, the inflammatory responses, and the antigens and mechanisms in these individuals that create the symptoms, can cause massive cell damage that lead to more severe disorders, syndromes, and even degenerative diseases of many types. Understanding how your body responds to inflammatory processes and determining the root cause of these reactions is vital to preventing sickness and disease. There are a countless number of people who needlessly suffer with pain and aggravating, sometimes debilitating symptoms, that could be prevented by some practical understanding and application.

It might surprise you to know that the simplest treatment can sometimes eliminate often even the most severe symptoms. I remember treating a patient who had brought her child with her to her appointment. She was sharing with me that her child had been having all sorts of health issues and seemed to be sick all of the time with colds, sore throats, and earaches. He also had an upset stomach (nausea) most all of the time.

While we were talking, she handed him a snack to keep him occupied. She gave him a small tomato, which seemed to be a healthy choice. When he bit into the tomato, it squirted out onto the side of his face a little bit because it was so juicy. When I looked back at the child less than a minute later I was startled to see a large red rash forming on his cheek. It was quite obvious the tomato was the culprit. She commented that he loved tomatoes and ate them almost every day. I advised her to remove them from his diet and explained to her that it is quite common to crave the very foods you are sensitive to. A few weeks later she returned to my office and was excited to report that her son had a miraculous change in his health status. No more runny nose, no colds, no sore throat or earaches. He was like a different child with his behavior. "From a tomato?" you may ask. Absolutely! I witnessed it with my own eyes. Most any physician who works with these types of food sensitivities has seen cases with similar presentations. The truth is, most people have no idea how common this phenomenon really is, especially in children.

Celiac disease is becoming more and more prevalent in our society. According to the Mayo Clinic more than half of the people who have celiac disease have signs and symptoms not associated with the digestive system, including: headaches, fatigue, joint pain, numbness and tingling in the hands and feet, problems with balance, cognitive impairment, anemia, osteoporosis, and itchy dermatitis.[1] Multiple studies discuss the different pain syndromes that can also manifest from the inflammatory response produced by this condition. If you ever have the blood tested and it returns positive for the deaminated gluten antibody (D.M.G.) then you are considered most likely to have celiac disease (an autoimmune disorder caused from extreme gluten sensitivity). The official diagnosis is made from doing a biopsy of the gut tissue to confirm it. If you are diagnosed with this condition you need to stay away from gluten containing foods. If you do, you should see many of your problems rapidly leaving your body. If anyone is suspect that they have it or if it runs in the family, they should be tested.

Have you ever heard of autism? Studies are now showing that when they take the autistic kids who are wheat-sensitive and gluten-sensitive off the gluten containing foods the results are nothing short of miraculous. Their little guts start to heal because they are taking away the offensive foods that produce cytokines that cross the blood-brain barrier and affect their brains.

In the epithelial linings of the lumen are white blood cells called **eosinophils**. They are very heavily populated around the lumen so that every time there is an immune response they produce histamine. **Histamine** is a nitrogenous compound that acts as a neurotransmitter in localized immune responses to modulate inflammatory responses. What does all that mean? This means that every time someone eats a food they are sensitive to, the eosinophils release histamine causing the gut to become inflamed. The diagnostic term for this condition is called **postprandial leukocytosis.** When individuals who have this condition eat foods they are sensitive to, those foods inflame the gut causing symptoms. This causes oxidation, inflammation, pain and discomfort, while disrupting the entire system and spreads throughout the body affecting multiple areas. The entire process is far more complex than this, but this is a basic explanation to better help to understand how this process works. Let's sum it up with a simple equation: Fix the gut + stop the inflammation = STOP THE PAIN.

STOP THE PAIN DIET

The Big 3: (REMOVE FROM THE DIET)

1) **Sugar** (all refined carbs, sweets, and avoid starchy foods like potatoes, as they convert directly into sugar.)

2) **Dairy** (any form of milk, yogurt, keifer, cream, etc.)

3) **Grains** (wheat, corn, oats, rice, all grains of any kind, or their by-products.)

These three foods (The Big Three) and their by-products are the most common general categories of food that cause immune activation and pro-inflammatory cytokine release in most people. This means they produce oxidation and inflammation in the body which in turn causes pain, swelling, fatigue, muscle soreness, sinus problems, allergies, inflammatory skin conditions, and destroys gut linings causing all kinds of digestive issues, just to name a few. These foods need to be avoided until the body has had time to heal itself. This can take on the average at least three to six months, and in some cases even longer. I've had multiple patients who have had their symptoms resolve by simply removing these foods from their diet alone. The common response to removing the "Big 3" are usually: more energy; better digestion with improved bowel function; resolved headaches, neck, back ,and joint pain; mental sharpness and clarity; and improved overall sense of well-being.

Anyone experiencing chronic pain and inflammation and/or autoimmune disease should consider removing these foods from the diet immediately. "Big 3 free"! This is an effective inexpensive way to get back on the road to recovery so your body can heal itself and STOP THE PAIN. These foods do not have to be permanently eliminated, but need to be removed until all of the inflammation is gone. After the body has recovered then some of these foods can be introduced.

Sinus Problems

People who have chronic sinus problems, tend to have antigens packed up in their sinuses. Considering the sinuses are dark, damp, and moist, make them a prime target for mold sensitivities and fungal infections. These types of infections typically are not affected by antibiotics and as a result are often left undetected and untreated. These hidden infections can initiate a chronic immune activation that causes the sinuses to inflame over time. Chronic sinusitis, recurrent infections, and other related sinus conditions are usually the result. Over time these continual immune activations can progress into more complex problems, and can even wind up causing the body to develop an **autoimmune response**. Depending on which

tissues are attacked determines what diagnosis is given. For example, if the A.N.A. blood test returns positive for the lupus antigen,
then the diagnosis is lupus. If the patient's lab results return positive
for rheumatoid factor and has anti-ccp antibodies present, rheumatoid arthritis is the diagnosis and so on. There's no lupus bug or
rheumatoid bug. These are autoimmune responses signifying an
over or continual stimulation of the immune system. Hidden infections, especially in the sinuses, can cause repetitive immune activations that can initiate immune responses that cause as well as promote autoimmune conditions. One simple approach in addressing
these responses is to treat the chronic infections to stop provoking
immune activation. When someone has chronic sinus problems and
is treated by our office, quite often we take two small cotton swabs,
dip them in a specially prepared silver protein solution, and place
them to the back of their sinuses. They are left in place for about
thirty to forty-five minutes to soak into the sinus cavities. Usually
within a few minutes thick globular mucous starts coming out of
the nostrils. The mucus expectorates cause those nasty antigens to
dump out and cleanse the sinuses. This allows your linings in the
sinus cavities to be free from the foreign invaders. Often the sinuses are so swollen that it's hard to get the swabs in because of the
amount of inflammation. Some of these people had been living with
these conditions for most of their lives and had no idea what was
causing the problem. The special silver protein solution preparation
used during the treatment also helps destroy the chronic fungal col-
onies and leaves a residue behind for several hours after completing
the treatment that continues to expectorate and cleanse the sinus. In
addition to the swabs, specially prepared iodine and colloidal silver-
based sprays are used daily in combination to make the treatment
more effective. After several treatments spread out over a few weeks
the sinuses usually clear up. The patients often report how amazing

it is to be able to breathe freely again.

This would be reward enough, but in a lot of those cases I actually discovered that their other inflammatory conditions seem to improve at the same time as the sinuses. Some of them had chronic pain for years and it simply disappeared after the sinuses were corrected. Many of my colleagues have experienced the same results. The sinuses are extremely vulnerable to inflammation and hidden infections, and need to be corrected in order to get the immune system to stop attacking the body.

Pollen is another antigen that provokes an immune activation. If you go outside and everything has a greenish yellow pollen all over it, then your sinuses will probably also have that same pollen coating on the inside of them after just a few breaths. Once you breathe it in it goes directly into the lungs and seeps into the bloodstream. If you take a blood spot sample and place it under a microscope, the pollen particles can actually be seen mixed in with the blood. That means histamine will be released on a systemic and not just a localized level. It now becomes a systemic problem in which the entire body becomes affected. One simple way to stop the body from responding with an immune reaction is to flush the sinuses with a **Nettie pot** before too many pollen molecules get into the bloodstream. Most stores that have pharmacies stock them and they're in abundance on the Internet. They are quick, easy, and convenient to use. They come with a small packet, which is basically a mixture of baking soda and salt, and should be mixed in distilled or at least filtered water. Flushing the sinuses with a Nettie pot a few times per day in the heavy pollen season can be a game changer for people who suffer from seasonal allergies. Adding some good old-fashioned Vick's salve in the nostrils at bedtime using a cotton swab also provides relief so you can get to sleep. Many people don't experience sinus symptoms from being exposed to dust or pollen, but instead get headaches, feel flu-like symptoms, or even have pain especially in areas where they have had problems in the past. Flushing out the sinuses can be a quick and sometimes immediate fix. Why wait until all of the histamine gets dispersed throughout your body, causing you to feel sluggish; to wake up in the morning and experience dizziness with the whole world spinning around you; to have migraine headaches; to have toxic, dark shiners under your eyes looking like your eyes are sunk in the back to the skull; to be so puffy and swollen that you can't get your rings off; or to feel like you have a pumpkin for a head. Some simple flushing can go a long way if you don't wait until it's too late.

Nebulizing Iodine and Colloidal Silver

Hidden infections are quite common and most people have no idea when they have one. Microorganisms like molds, viruses, parasites, and even certain bacterias, can find their way into places where the body cannot fight them properly. Places like the intestines, teeth, and especially the sinuses can be targets for these types of infections. The sinuses are dark, damp, and often stagnant which make them a prime candidate for fungal and/or microbial infections. If someone suspects they have one of these hidden infections, nebulizing **nascent iodine** or colloidal silver can be quite effective in correcting this problem. Nascent iodine is simply a form of iodine that's already converted to usable iodine in the body. Most iodine that's added to the diet has to be converted from inorganic to organic bound, which is the kind that is used by the body. Regular store bought iodine (inorganically bound) is not recommended for nebulizing. Nascent iodine, on the other hand, is an excellent form to use as it is already converted and destroys these microbes on contact. Six to eight drops mixed in 2-3 ml of sterile saline solution or sterile water is typically a good starting dose. The dose can be given at a higher dose, but as with all nebulization, should be medically supervised. I personally like to remove the mouthpiece and gently insert the opening of the cap that covers the bowl into the base of the nostril and breathe normally, alternating between nostrils after taking two breaths in each nostril, until the bowl is empty. This can be done one time per day, two to three times per week if tolerated well. Sometimes it may cause a slight burning sensation, especially if the sinuses are really irritated. This is usual and only lasts for a few seconds. If it's too uncomfortable, stop the treatment and use colloidal silver instead. Of course anyone with iodine sensitivities should never nebulize iodine or take iodine supplements. Colloidal silver can also be used and is a little less harsh so it can be used more frequently and daily. The colloidal silver doesn't need to be diluted, just add two to three ml to the nebulizer and follow the same technique. The treatment is soothing, simple, and is usually quite effective. Colloidal silvers can actually be purchased in a nose spray bottle and used several times per day if needed. However, most people usually don't administer enough to give good results. Ten to fifteen sprays in each nostril is usually a safe, effective dose, three to four times per day for a week or so. Alternating from one solution to the other during the treatments can also be a good strategy if someone isn't responding as well as expected. If these hidden infections are not eliminated, they can cause chronic cytokine responses that provoke immune responses that lead to the inflammatory cascade. The end result is usually pain, soreness, and discomfort. Destroying these microbes can result in stopping this process allowing the body to recover, repair, and rejuvenate itself. Once the microbes are gone the cytokine response should stop and the pain and suffering should be over. Many times adding treatments like these can be the game changer for breaking the chronic pain cycle and helping you to STOP THE PAIN.

The Immune System

The immune system is amazing. It has different types of cells that are released - Th1's, Th2's, CD4's, CD8's, Th17's, killer cells, B cells, T cells, just to name a few. These are different types of immune cells including macrophages that come on the scene to attack and devour the invaders once they make it into your body.

There are a lot of invaders on the food that you are eating every day. Most people think after food is rinsed off its okay; however, even though you rinse it and wash it, there are still a lot of bacteria, molds and their by-products, and a host of other microorganisms that find their way into your body. We eat, drink, and even breathe them in on a regular basis. We touch them and then they transfer from hand-to-mouth. This is called **autoinoculation**. When someone sneezes or coughs beside you, the contaminated particles are nebulized, inhaled into the lungs, and are deposited directly into the bloodstream. We cannot make the world go away nor hide from it. The fact is, things are constantly invading our body, and thank God we are equipped with an immune activation system, that once the invaders are detected and reported, then the body sends an army to greet it. Once the army attacks, there will be damage reported on a localized level. If the process is quick and it is painless, the person may not even experience any symptoms at all. These types of encounters are happening continually, occurring each and every day of our lives. This is actually how we acquire our immunity making them stronger and more resistant to infections. Once the body develops an antibody to destroy a pathogen, it records it in the internal pharmacy. If that pathogen ever presents again, the body already has the weapon in its arsenal to use against it.

This process continues and if, for some reason, the invaders get a little more aggressive, the immune system will activate and dispatch a more aggressive attack in response. The dendritic cells are the ones that inspect whatever enters the body and, if necessary, reports them by releasing cytokines. A cytokine is just a messenger protein molecule that is sent through the bloodstream to report to the brain and/or to the parts of the immune system, depending on what area that needs to be notified. These cytokines are inflammatory by nature, which means they may provoke an immune response. The more cytokines released, the more aggressive the response.

Remember, if you roll your ankle, the first sign of any cellular damage, especially from a traumatic injury, is inflammation. Swelling! When you have something that is producing collateral damage, swelling and inflammation will follow. What happens to your jaw when you have a swollen tooth? It swells and becomes sore and painful. What happens when something gets infected? It inflames at the site of the infected area causing pain and discomfort. Wherever there is a hidden infection anywhere in the body, it will provoke an inflammatory cytokine response causing an immune activation.

When something is inflamed for a longer period of time, there is also a spreading of cellular damage in those peripheral tissues as the result of the prolonged effects of the inflammation. This also continues to stimulate this vicious cycle of pain and inflammation causing it to spread throughout the body. This can severely deplete the body's energy system and lower the metabolic rate by affecting the hypothalamus, thyroid, and adrenal system. Almost all stressors share the activation of the hypothalamic-pituitary-adrenocortical axis and of the sympathetic nervous system with subsequent onset of inflammation and oxidative stress.[2] If these glandular systems become deficient in function it can cause a chain reaction of events that take place throughout the body causing severe disruption of the body systems.

Opportunists

Once the metabolism starts to slow down, the gut function is one of the first systems to suffer the effects. This process slows down the transit time in the digestive tract, allows microorganisms to grow unchallenged and become very well established in the entire gut. If these bad bugs go untreated, they can cause a lot of symptoms, not only in the gut but also throughout the entire body. The most common of these fall into four main categories:

1. Parasites

2. Yeast

3. Virus

4. Bacteria

These energy vampires literally feed from the nutrients and energy produced by your body causing fatigue, irritation, and all types of aches and pains. They not only rob the body of its precious resources, but they also can produce toxicity and other poisons that wreak havoc in the body. Along with the bug overgrowth, the slowed function causes lack of proper digestion, which, in turn, causes a problem with proper assimilation and absorption of vital nutrients. These deficiencies lead to fatigue, irritation, and all types of aches and pains.

Autoimmune Disorders

Hidden infections, chronic repetitive immune activations from sensitivities, and/or toxicities from pollutants, individually or combined, can produce autoimmune responses that can further progress into autoimmune disorders. For example, almost every patient I have treated that has had breast augmentations has also had some form of autoimmune response as a result. Some of them lie dormant and only produce little to no symptoms. However, a larger number seem to manifest as inflammatory and/or metabolic disorders. The immune system and the thyroid seem to be particularly sensitive to the implants, silicone, or saline. I have had multiple patients who developed conditions such as rheumatoid arthritis, lupus, or fibromyalgia shortly after having breast augmentations. If you've already had the surgery don't panic. If the body is treated properly the toxic condition can usually be improved without having to have them removed. However, I have seen cases where it was necessary in order to stop the reactions. The object here is to help you to identify the causes that may be initiating the symptoms you are experiencing. There are so many people suffering from autoimmune disorders that have no idea that these are potential causes for problems they are experiencing. Mercury amalgam fillings in teeth, cosmetic implants, etc., or any other toxin to the body that's implanted, ingested, inhaled, or absorbed can initiate immune responses that can lead to autoimmune disorders and diseases. When someone is diagnosed with an autoimmune disorder, **four things** should be considered for treatment at the moment the diagnosis is made.

1. Test for **gut and systemic sensitivities** and treat them.

2. Evaluate for **potential toxicity** and treat it.

3. Search for **hidden infections** and treat them.

4. Control **oxidative and inflammatory responses** while treating the other conditions.

Thyroid

"Help me! I'm swollen, bloated, pale, puffy, plump, and everything hurts." Sound familiar? If this sounds like you or someone you know, start smiling because help is on the way. I wish I had a dollar for every time I've heard these complaints in clinical practice. These would be considered by most to be classic symptoms of an underactive thyroid gland. The **thyroid** is a butterfly shaped gland that sits towards the front at the base of the neck slightly below the Adam's apple. One of its primary functions is producing iodine-containing hormones that increase the body's basal metabolic rate. These hormones also influence the system in many other important ways, such as: appetite, absorption in the gut, intestinal motility, stimulate the breakdown of fats, and affect mood and mental function ,to name a few. The thyroid gland is involved both directly and indirectly with the balance and regulation of hormones throughout the system. If its function is increased or decreased, serious disruptions can occur systemically affecting almost every other system in the body.

One of the most common thyroid conditions is referred to as **hypothyroidism** (an underactive thyroid). This denotes an underactive thyroid gland that cannot maintain an adequate level of thyroid hormone causing a decline in body function, especially in the metabolism and gut. When gut function is compromised, all function is compromised. If digestion, assimilation and absorption of essential nutrients, and proper disposal of waste products are compromised in any way, the entire body is compromised as well. This is exactly what takes place when someone's thyroid becomes underactive. The devastating effects can be seen even in the early stages of dysfunction and if it goes untreated it can be potentially life-threatening. The symptoms manifest in a way that presents as if the body is breaking down because that's exactly what is happening. Everything from digestion to hormone imbalance to chronic pain starts to occur, and the combined problems seem to amplify the symptom profile.

Many people who have this condition are not aware of it because it can have a very slow and gradual onset. Some people just think they are getting older. Still others feel that they are just stressed out. The truth is both of those scenarios may be true, but they are not the primary reason for the pain and suffering. An underactive thyroid gland is far more common than most people are aware of. When treated properly the patients usually recover nicely and when managed properly typically continue to respond very well to treatment. The important question to ask is, "Are you suffering from an underactive thyroid condition?"

Quickly take this survey. If you have three or more of these symptoms, there's a high probability that you have an underactive thyroid.

Thyroid Survey:

- ☐ Poor bowel habits like constipation or poor quality stools

- ☐ Fatigue and low energy

- ☐ Low sex drive and loss of motivation

- ☐ Slowed metabolism

- ☐ Hair loss and thinning (especially showing up in the shower drain)

- ☐ Pale, dry skin

- ☐ Brittle nails and/or hair

- ☐ Muscle aches and soreness

- ☐ Anxiety and/or depression

If you have these symptoms you should have your thyroid evaluated immediately. Simple and complete blood testing can be used to diagnose this condition so it can be properly treated. If you are having your thyroid tested insist that your physician includes the **free T4, free T3, T.P.A.,T.P.O., reverse T3 and TSH** when they order the blood work, or the underlying problem cannot be addressed and most likely the symptom will get treated but the cause will continue to cause long-term imbalance. If you do not have access or can't afford lab testing, there is a simple and free test that can be done in the comfort of your own home called a **Barnes test**. I monitor all of my thyroid patients using this test as one of their metabolic indicators. It requires that the axillary (arm pit) temperature be taken before arising each morning at the same time each day. It should be done for thirty days and the results recorded each time the temperature is taken. The old-fashioned glass thermometers are the most accurate. The normal axillary core body temperature should be 97.6, exactly 1 degree less than when taken under the tongue. Individuals who have an underactive thyroid will have core temperatures much lower than normal. It's not uncommon at all to review findings recorded in the low 90s. My experience has been that the lower the temperature, the worse the condition. I can't say this is an absolute for everyone but it has been a consistent finding in my office. Sometimes the blood work returns normal, yet it's obvious the patient's thyroid is deficient. This condition is referred to as a subclinical hypothyroid disorder. The Barnes test is a good option to use to confirm this. If the body's temperatures are low, then there's a high likelihood the thyroid function is impaired, even if the blood work is normal. If the temperatures are normal and so is the blood work, then there's the highest probability that the thyroid is not the problem. Below is a list of causes that explains some reasons for why the thyroid could appear to be normal yet its function still be impaired. This list is a **five-point evaluation** that should be considered in the overall diagnosis and management of a thyroid patient.

Feeding a patient thyroid hormone, natural or synthetic, is only addressing one spoke in a much larger metabolic process and does not correct the true underlying problem. If the evaluation reveals one or more of these causes to be the problem, they can usually be corrected and never have to be prescribed thyroid hormone.

Five reasons for basic thyroid blood tests to appear normal when the thyroid is clearly the problem:

(5 point evaluation)

1) **Autoimmune dysfunction** (sensitivity, toxicity, and/or hidden infection)

Thyroid (Hashimoto's Thyroiditis Disease)

Hashimoto's disease is a condition in which the immune system attacks the thyroid. It is classified as an autoimmune disorder that is often missed because routine T4 and TSH levels sometimes return normal. Thyroid antibodies (TPO, TPA) can be tested with a simple blood test to evaluate for this condition. If someone's blood test returns positive, they are considered to have autoimmune thyroid disease, more commonly referred to as Hashimoto's Thyroiditis Disease. How does this condition occur?

Anything that provokes the gut lining, such as an antigen or microbe, causes the body to release **pro-inflammatory cytokines** (protein messengers that trigger inflammation). When I send a patient for a food sensitivity panel, ninety-six foods are tested. When the results return, it reveals the foods the person is sensitive to, which means every time they eat those foods, it produces an immune response in their gut. The gut has cells that act like little sentinels, they are little guard cells called **dendritic cells**; and they are dispersed throughout the lumen of the gut. They have little tentacles, sort of like an octopus, that push up in the lumen feeling around for foreign invading substances. If they feel a particular food product and determine that it should not be there, the first thing they do is label it. "This one is okay," or "This one is **stranger—danger.**" Once a stranger — danger gets labeled, the immune system releases macrophages, B cells, natural killer cells, and here comes the cavalry. They are looking for the ones that are labeled "stranger-danger." This causes an internal war, because when a meal is full of stranger-dangers, the food disrupts normal function of the gut.

Let's say someone had a stomach virus, and while the system was fighting the infection they ate a carrot. When things like viruses get mixed with food particles, sometimes they get labeled as a threat to the body as well. If in the above scenario the carrot gets mixed in with the virus, it may get labeled "stranger-danger" as a threat along with the virus. This is what sets up the sensitivities to foods. Let's say three weeks later, the virus is gone, the immune system has successfully defeated it, and you eat some carrots. It goes to your gut and the dendritic cell recognizes it because it is labeled "Stranger-danger." It then reports it to the immune system, initiates an immune response, and starts attacking your gut again. The same symptoms return as when the stomach virus was present except this time, there is no infection. The carrot provokes a full-blown immune response in the body. If they continue over and over there's another problem that occurs. There is a process called **molecular mimicry**. It occurs when body tissues get labeled along with the foreign invading substances and gets labeled "stranger-danger" as well. When the gut continues to get bombarded by immune responses the actual gut lining cells (their amino acid sequence) get labeled as stranger-danger.

When these immune responses are continually activated they can migrate to other parts of the body. The thyroid in particular is vulnerable to repeated attacks because the thyroid tissue often gets labeled as stranger-danger as well. The problem with this condition is every time there is an immune response, like from a cold, the flu, or a sensitive food, the body goes back to the same areas and repeats the attack because of molecular mimicry of those tissues. This means if you have been treated for Hashimoto thyroiditis in the past you may have stabilized from that condition. Two weeks from now you get the flu and when your body has an immune response to the flu bug, it also attacks the thyroid again. Boom! Your thyroid goes haywire and your physician has to readjust your medications to bring it back to balance.

Worse yet, if you eat the carrot that the body developed a sensitivity to, it provokes an immune response and the thyroid gets attacked again. That's why no one should ever get their thyroid tested on a day when they have any type of sickness or allergic response. The test results will become skewed as a result of the insult to the thyroid. The gut is usually the culprit for setting up most of these types of reactions and should be treated to repair the linings and to restore the microbiome. If not, the thyroid will continue to re-exacerbate every time there is an immune response. When the thyroid gets attacked it can then overstimulate the production of thyroid hormones and produce a hyperthyroid (an overactive thyroid). This can even have symptoms and consequences worse than the hypothyroid condition. Individuals who are diagnosed with this condition are recommended to completely remove all gluten from the diet. This is a precaution to prevent an immune response from causing a repeat attack on the thyroid. Hidden infections in the teeth, sinuses, and other places in the body also cause these same immune activations. These underlying causes must be addressed and treated. If not, this terrible metabolic seesaw will continue to get worse. There are many people out there today who are suffering from autoimmune conditions or Hashimoto's thyroiditis disease and have no idea that sensitivities from the gut and/or hidden infections can be the root cause of their disorder.

2) Halogen toxicity

Halogen toxicity occurs when the body substitutes the right form of iodine with another molecule that prevents the hormone from being active. Iodine is a vital micronutrient required at all stages of life, fetal life and early childhood being the most critical phases of requirement. Diet is the sole source of iodine, which in turn is dependent upon the iodine content of water and soil. Iodine is metabolized in the human body through a series of stages involving the hypothalamus, pituitary, thyroid gland, and blood. The thyroid gland constructs the thyroid hormone by combining the amino acid **L-tyrosine** with **organic bound iodine**. Iodine is listed in the periodic table as a **halogen**. There are other halogens (**fluorine, bromine,** and **chlorine**) that humans come in contact with, that are very close in size and structure as iodine. If the body is deficient in iodine, the body will use one of these other halogens to bind with the L-tyrosine in order to make thyroid hormone. The problem is, although structurally it looks like the normal hormone, it's not biologically active. This means it can't do what the body needs it to do to maintain a normal metabolism. There are many cases when patients have all of the symptoms of being deficient in thyroid hormone but go to their physicians and have their thyroid hormone levels tested and the tests come back normal. How can this be? The reason is there are normal levels of hormone but it's not active because it's missing the proper iodine content. There is fluoride in our toothpaste and water sources, bromine in our breads and buns, and chlorine in our pools and showers. People don't even realize the fact that they are nebulizing chlorine and fluorine directly into their bloodstream every time they take a shower because these halogens are in our water. Is it any wonder that so many people have metabolic syndromes and symptoms of an underactive thyroid? The good news is that if you are suffering from this condition, it is easily corrected. In order to get rid of the toxic halogen imposters in the system, the iodine deficiency must be corrected. Taking the right amount of the correct type of iodine (prolamine or nascent iodine) will correct this deficiency in just a few weeks. Organic bound iodine has a stronger affinity to bind than the other halogens, so when it's added back to the system it literally kicks off the wrong halogens and replaces it with the iodine, causing it to convert to the active form. Once the hormone quality is restored the metabolic function also returns to normal.

3) Vitamin D deficiency and/or receptor resistance problem.

Vitamin D is commonly known as the "sunshine vitamin." The truth is, however, this often-misunderstood "vitamin" is actually a **prohormone**. Prohormones are substances that the body converts to a hormone. In fact, unlike other vitamins, only a portion of the vitamin D that the body needs comes from food (such as dairy, meat, and eggs), and the rest the body makes for itself. There are some that will argue that vitamin D is not a prohormone but instead a **prehormone**. Neither viewpoint changes the outcome of what vitamin D is capable of accomplishing in the system.

Vitamin D obtained from sun exposure, food, and supplements is biologically inert and must undergo two hydroxylations in the body for activation. The first occurs in the liver and converts **vitamin D to 25-hydroxyvitamin D [25(OH)D]**, also known as **calcidiol**. The second occurs primarily in the kidney and forms the physiologically active **1,25-dihydroxyvitamin D [1,25(OH)2D]**, also known as **calcitriol**.[3]

Vitamin D has its effects by binding to a protein (called the **vitamin D receptor**). This receptor is present in nearly every cell and affects many different body processes.

Refined sugar is a highly inflammatory substance in the human body when taken in excess. Chronic indulgence of sweets causes overactive insulin responses that over time blunt a variety of receptors causing conditions such as insulin resistance. Other receptors are also affected by this process because of the amount of inflammation and oxidation being generated in the system. The vitamin D receptor is one of these that suffers from this condition. If the receptors aren't converting, then vitamin D levels cannot normalize and the body will experience symptoms as a result.

There seems to be a craze right now that's causing everyone to take incredibly high doses of vitamin D because their blood tests are showing that they are deficient. Once again you can't just look at one level and make an assumption about what the treatment needs to be. In some cases, ramping up the vitamin D will correct the problem. However, in many cases it is only part of the problem. Sometimes other nutrients like **K1** and **K2** are needed for conversion in order for the levels to normalize. Yet for this discussion, there's a bigger problem to address, and that is the condition when the Vitamin D receptors are not converting properly and therefore doesn't make the conversion necessary to make vitamin D fully functional. In order for vitamin D to do its job completely, it has to be converted into its active form. If the receptors are blunted and have become resistant, then they don't convert properly and it results in deficiency. The only way to know is to test both the **1,25 dihydroxycholecalciferol** (physiological active form) and the **25 hydroxycholecalciferol**. A simple blood test from a physician can find out if you have this conversion problem. If the receptors are resistant there are compounds in nature that science has shown to improve this resistance and allows the proper conversions to take place. **Resveratrol, green tea catechins, alpha lipoic acid,** and **curcumin,** when taken in their proper doses, have all demonstrated positive clinical results for restoring this conversion process. There are others but these are some of the most common used to treat this condition naturally. Before jumping on the bandwagon of the latest vitamin D fad, why not have your levels tested and find the true root of the problem.

Vitamin D is not only important for proper calcium absorption but research now shows a direct correlation between vitamin D levels and thyroid function. Brazilian researchers conducted a study focused on the prevalence of vitamin D insufficiency and the link to thyroid size, function, and autoimmunity markers in Hashimoto's thyroid patients. The researchers concluded that low vitamin D is involved in the disease process that causes Hashimoto's thyroiditis, and that vitamin D and autoimmune thyroid disease are linked.[4] Vitamin D supplementation also has shown promise as a way to help treat thyroid disease. In the Greek study, for example, the Hashimoto thyroiditis patients who were deficient in vitamin D took 1,200 to 4,000 international units (IU) of vitamin D every day for four months, after which time they had significantly lower levels of anti-thyroid antibodies.[5] In yet another study, people with hypothyroidism who took extra vitamin D supplements for 12 weeks had improvements in blood levels of thyroid stimulating hormone (although the extra D did not affect levels of the actual thyroid hormones triiodothyronine, T3, and thyroxine, T4).[6]

The research clearly suggests that maintaining normal levels of vitamin D plays a crucial role in treating and correcting thyroid problems.

4) Deiodinase activation problem.

In order for the thyroid hormone to be converted to its active form it has to be activated. **Activation** occurs by conversion of the prohormone **thyroxine (T4)** to the active hormone **triiodothyronine**

(T3) through the removal of an iodine atom on the outer ring. To accurately assess thyroid function, it must be understood that deiodinase enzymes are what control cellular thyroid activity and determine intracellular activation and deactivation of thyroid hormones.

There are three main enzymes that regulate the control of thyroid hormone to either activate it or inactivate it. **D1, D2, and D3** are the three diodinase enzymes that regulate this control. D1 and D2 enzymes convert the T4 hormone into active T3 hormone. The D3 enzyme reduces thyroid activity by converting T4 the anti-thyroid reverse T3 (reverse T3). In order for the hormone to make the thyroid hormone active or useful, it is dependent on **selenium**. One particular study done on mice demonstrated that selenium deficiency adversely affects thyroid hormone metabolism and decreases 5 prime deiodination of T4.[7] If someone is selenium deficient the hormone cannot be activated and the patient can start to experience symptoms of a thyroid imbalance. Selenium is an antioxidant that protects the cells from oxidative damage, especially in the heart, so people who have high levels of oxidation or are under very stressful loads fall prey to selenium deficiency. Meats and nuts are rich in selenium and people who are on vegan diets need to make sure they get plenty from vegetable sources or supplementation. Selenium plays a significant role in thyroid hormone function and needs to be considered for those who are dealing with thyroid problems.

5) **Triclosan** is a disrupter of the thyroid gland and is one of the most common ingredients that's found in antibacterial soaps. A survey done in 2007 showed that 76 percent of commercial soaps contained triclosan. Triclosan works by disrupting a critical enzyme (called ENR) that bacteria use in the synthesis of fatty acids. When ENR is disrupted by triclosan, the bacteria can no longer form or repair cell walls, resulting in the death of the cell. Humans do not

have the ENR enzyme, so it appeared that triclosan would not have any harmful effects. Triclosan, like most harmful chemicals, can be absorbed into the bloodstream through the skin. A 2007 study done on over 2,500 participants showed that 75 percent had biologically significant levels of triclosan in their urine.[8]

The skin is the largest organ in the body, and most of the chemicals in shampoos and soaps are most likely being absorbed in some quantity through it. Triclosan is no exception to the rule and research actually reveals certain health problems that this chemical is causing as a result of it getting into the system.

Triclosan has a few of the same key structural chemical similarities as triiodothyronine (T3, the active form of thyroid hormone). This similarity seems to cause a significant amount of disruption in the production of normal thyroid hormone levels.

Studies have demonstrated that exposure to triclosan produces a dose-dependent decrease in serum levels of both T3 and T4 thyroid hormones.[9]

These thyroid hormones are a primary regulator of metabolic activity throughout the body — so reducing levels of T3 and T4 in the body could lead to weight gain, decreased energy levels, depression, and the other symptoms commonly associated with hypothyroidism.

Triclosan has also been shown to have estrogenic activities in the body. This can only add to the slowed fat metabolism and weight gain potential in males and females. It certainly could make things worse for men who already have low testosterone levels. Clearly research supports the understanding that these antibacterial soaps have potential to disrupt the normal function of the thyroid gland and its ability to produce normal levels of hormone that are vital in order to have a good metabolism and maintain optimal health. It certainly appears as though they seem to cause more harm than good. The takeaway message is simple, **"Stop using antibacterial soaps."**

Thyroid Recovery

According to the American Association of Clinical Endocrinologists (AACE), thyroid disease is more common than diabetes or heart disease and affects as many as 30 million Americans. Recent news stories have also linked thyroid issues to both **weight gain** and **infertility**, and this media attention is finally starting to bring the conversation about thyroid dysfunction to the forefront. This is such an important finding for those who want to have children but have been told they have infertility problems. The thyroid should be one of the first things evaluated for those who are dealing with this problem. However, the basic routine thyroid testing will more than likely overlook the five problems just pointed out. If your physician won't consider doing these evaluations, then find one who will. There are plenty of good physicians out there who will put their ego in check and at least consider what's best for their patient. Thyroid problems can be contributors to so many pain syndromes and disorders from chronic fatigue to fibromyalgia. From hormone imbalances to the inability to lose weight, poor digestion and elimination, to even depression, all or any of these problems can be the result of an imbalance of thyroid function. The five-point evaluation may be able to reveal a problem that's been hiding in your system that has been overlooked or possibly even misdiagnosed.

Adrenal dysfunction and cortisol overload (positive Ragland test) also play an important role in the ability to correct a thyroid imbalance. If this is the case, supporting the glands with targeted nutrients along with restoring proper electrolyte balance, can help to fortify any deficiencies caused by this condition. There are many people who are also suffering with anxiety and/or depression as the result of thyroid dysfunction. This is probably more accurately a problem with **suppression** that's causing symptoms of depression. When the metabolic processes are slowed due to an underactive thyroid, gut function, hormone imbalance, as well as neurotransmitter, disruption can occur. When thyroid function is "suppressed," one of the classic symptoms is that the mental state becomes "depressed." S.S.R.I. drugs may not be the best choice for this situation, but instead the thyroid function needs to be restored. Hopefully the information provided will shed some light on how to resolve any thyroid issues you may be dealing with.

Mitochondrial Dysfunction

There are organelles in the cells that are called **mitochondria**. They are often referred to as the powerhouse of the cells because that is where the energy is produced that runs the body processes. In order for these little factories to produce the energy that the body requires, they must have certain vitamins, minerals, and cofactors (helpers). If they become deprived of these vital substances the energy levels begin to decline. Energy production in mitochondria is absolutely essential to sustain life and it plays a part in anything from physical strength to endurance and alertness. Even a slight decrease in the production of energy from mitochondria can quickly manifest as physical weakness, pain and soreness, inability to concentrate (brain fog), and fatigue. The mitochondria and their function are part of what determines the quality of our life. They are in every cell of the body. When you get prolonged inflammation and pain over time, it eventually will lead to mitochondrial damage. This causes an energy crisis in the body and impairs the rate at which healing needs to occur.

Every time there is an immune activation, there is a demand on the energy system and the deficit gets worse many times resulting in pain syndromes. That explains why so many people with chronic pain usually have hidden infections as well, and because everyone is so focused on the pain, the underlying cause goes unnoticed. The chronic and continual damage from oxidation and inflammation combined with the immune activation from the underlying hidden infection adds to this energy deficit to the point where the person may experience extreme fatigue, physical weakness, and chronic pain. The good news is, the mitochondria can repair, regenerate, and reproduce themselves to recover from this assault. This process is called **mitochondrial biogenesis** and can be defined as the growth and division of preexisting mitochondria. Mitochondria are direct descendants of an a-protobacteria endosymbiont that became established in a host cell. Owing to their bacterial origin, mitochondria have their own genome and can autoreplicate.[10] Reactivating and maintaining mitochondrial function should be a top priority for anyone who has been suffering from debilitating pain, devastating energy loss, and/ or a chronic poor state of health and can't seem to recover.

> **" Reactivating and maintaining mitochondrial function should be a top priority for anyone who has been suffering from debilitating pain, devastating energy loss, and/ or a chronic poor state of health and can't seem to recover. "**

There are specific nutrients needed for the mitochondria to make energy:

1. B-complex, the full range of B vitamins, but especially B1, B2, and B3

2. Magnesium (a mineral antioxidant)

3. Zinc (a mineral antioxidant)

4. Manganese (a mineral antioxidant)

5. Glutathione (the master antioxidant)

6. NAD (derived from Vitamin B3).

7. Alpha Lipoic Acid (an antioxidant)

8. Carnitine (metabolizes fat)

9. CoQ10 (protects mitochondria from damage)

The **Mitochondrial (Energy) Reactivation Protocol (MRP) is** designed to provide the body with the right activity, nutritional support, dietary solutions, and lifestyle choices needed to repair and restore normal function to the mitochondrial system that provides energy for the body. **Less energy = Less repair, More energy = More repair.** Combining with H.I.I.T. training, prayer and meditation, and supporting the adrenal system is a well-rounded approach to getting the mitochondria back to an optimal state of function. It's kind of like recharging the batteries in the cells and fixing the alternator both at the same time.

MITOCHONDRIAL (Energy) REACTIVATION PROTOCOL

Adrenal Support has the full range of B vitamins and other natural ingredients that research shows work as cofactors to assist in mito-chondrial function and support adrenal function. Both of these systems work together to generate and maintain optimal energy levels.

ALA/ALC (alpha lipoic acid/acetyl L carnitine) research shows it helps to reverse mitochondrial dysfunction and helps promote the fat burning metabolism to produce high-quality energy for a higher energy yield.

MITOGEN (converted and unconverted CoQ10) research shows CoQ10 helps protect the mitochondria from oxidative damage making them more efficient at producing energy. It also contains calcium pyruvate to assist the body in producing energy more efficiently.

MINSORB contains highly absorbable minerals, especially magnesium, zinc, and manganese, that research shows play a significant role in optimizing mitochondrial metabolism. Remember back in science class when the teacher put two wires in a bowl full of water and put a light bulb in at the other end of the bowl. The light bulb would not light up when the current was turned on. However, at the moment the teacher added minerals to the water, the light bulb would start to glow. The more minerals that were added to the water, the brighter the light would glow until it finally reached full capacity. That's how minerals work in the body. They help to recharge the system helping us function at full capacity.

H.I.I.T training has been proven to enhance mitochondrial function. (See detailed instruction on p.210.) A study published in *Cell Metabolism* found that exercise — and in particular high-intensity interval training in aerobic exercises such as biking and walking — caused cells to make more proteins for their energy-producing mitochondria and their protein-building ribosomes, effectively stopping aging at the cellular level. Short interval training at a high intensity can be utilized by most any style of exercise from doing push-ups and jumping jacks to riding a bike, or jogging and sprinting. You don't have to buy any equipment or pay for a gym membership to do this style of workout. Anyone can do it at any entry level of fitness, from the most out of shape to the Olympic athlete. The workout routine can be constructed for anyone, at any age, for only six or more minutes per day.

> **"The time and money you spend investing in your body will ultimately yield the highest returns."**

Do this protocol for at least three months minimum in order to reestablish a better quality of energy and endurance. "The time and money you spend investing in your body will ultimately yield the highest returns."

ENZYME THERAPY

When foods are triggering immune responses in the gut, the end result can be sickness and pain. The cytokines released by the gut in response to the offending foods are made up of proteins. When **digestive enzymes** are given at a clinical dose, they digest the protein complexes that the cytokine messengers are composed of and therefore stops the cytokine response so the immune system doesn't respond. This can be a highly effective treatment for people who have a large number of food sensitivities. The people who suffer from this response usually have no idea why they are feeling bad and suffering from pain. If you suspect that you may be one of those who have this problem, simply ask your physician to run an IgG/IgA ninety-six foods panel and by one simple blood draw you can know if this is a part or all of your problem. If the panel comes back positive, then stay off of the offending foods and add L- glutamine at twenty-five to thirty grams in sixteen ounces of water per day for two to three months. This will help restore the damage done to the gut from the chronic inflammatory responses. After eliminating the offending foods for a couple of weeks and taking the L-glutamine, start adding back the lower sensitivity foods one at a time taking a few digestive enzyme capsules with those foods to help digest any cytokines. Take your pulse before you add back the sensitive food and take it again five minutes after you eat it and take the enzymes. If the pulse stays the same then the body is probably accepting the food. If the pulse rises higher than five beats per minute then you may have to eliminate that food for a couple weeks longer. Slowly add back the sensitive foods adding one every few days each time taking enzymes with it. This is a really good way to desensitize the gut to the foods you've been sensitive to. If you are allergic to any foods, you should stay away from those foods and consult your physician about possibly carrying an epipen as a precaution.

FIX#3: Pain Stoppers

- Identify any food sensitivities and avoid those foods.

- Remove the big 3 from your diet (Big 3 free).

- Supplement with L glutamine (25-30 grams) daily in order to assist the body in healing the damaged epithelial linings.

- Correct any sinus problems with nebulized iodine and/or colloidal silver spray.

- Address any thyroid and/or adrenal issues and supplement by adding targeted nutrients (such as iodine, L-tyrosine, etc.) as needed.

- Begin the MITOCHONDRIAL REACTIVATION PROTOCOL. (Add MITOGEN, ALA/ALC, MINSORB, ADRENAL SUPPORT, and start doing H.I.I.T. exercises.)

- Add enzymes to each meal to improve digestion and reduce inflammatory cytokines.

Chapter 8: Immune Responses

1. Celiac disease; mayoclinic.org: overview.

2. Antioxid. Redox Signal. 28, 735–740.Published Online:20 Mar 2018https://doi.org/10.1089/ars.2017.7488.

3. Institute of Medicine, Food and Nutrition Board. Dietary Reference Intakes for Calcium and Vitamin D. Washington, DC: National Academy Press, 2010.

4. Chen, G. et. al. "Serum Vitamin D3 Level in Patients with Autoimmune Thyroid Diseases," "Abstracts from the American Thyroid Association," *Thyroid*, Volume 24, Supplement 1, 2014, Poster 18, October 2014.

5. Mazokopakis E E, Papadom Anolaki MG, Tsekaras KC, Evangelopoulas AD, Kotsiris DA, Tzortzinas AA. Is vitamin D related to pathogenesis and treatment of Hashimoto's thyroiditis? Hell J Nucl Med. 2015 Sep-Dec;18(3):222-7.

6. Yasin Simseki, Ilkay Cakir, Mikail Yemtmis, Oguzhan Sitka Dizdar, Ferhat Gokay. Dept of endocrinology and metabolism, Kayseri Training and Research Hospital, Kayseri Turkey. Dept of Internal Medicine, Bagcilar Training and Research Hospital, Istanbul, Turkey. Dept of Internal Medicine, Okayseri Training and Research Hospital, Kayseri, Turkey.

7. J R Arthur, F Nicol, and G J Beckett Biochem J. Hepatic iodothyronine 5'-deiodinase. The role of selenium. 1990 Dec 1; 272(2): 537–540.

8. Urinary Concentrations of Triclosan in the U.S. Population: 2003–2004 Antonia M. Calafat, Xiaoyun Ye, [...], and Larry L. Needham.

9. Crit Rev Toxicol. 2014 Jul;44(6):535-55. doi: 10.3109/10408444.2014.910754. Epub 2014 Jun. Critical analysis of endocrine disruptive activity of triclosan and its relevance to human exposure through the use of personal care products. Witorsch RJ1. Environ Toxicol Pharmacol. 2007 Sep;24(2):194-7. doi: 10.1016/j.etap.2007.04.008. Epub 2007 Apr 27. Short-term in vivo exposure to the water contaminant triclosan: Evidence for disruption of thyroxine. Crofton KM1, Paul KB, Devito MJ, Hedge JM.

10. Regulation of mitochondrial biogenesis François R. Jornayvaz and Gerald I. Shulman Essays Biochem. 2010;47:10.1042/bse 0470069 author manuscript.

SECTION

4

INFLAMMATION

CHAPTER NINE

Inflammation
Natural Anti-inflammatories

What drives pain? Inflammation! What motivates you to do something about a problem? Pain! What makes people desperate for relief to the point they will take all sorts of toxic and even highly addictive medications or do radical procedures that can leave them maimed and handicapped if the attempts fail? Pain and inflammation!

Pain and Inflammation, the Dynamic Duo

The very things that warn someone damage is occurring and initiate the healing process have also been the target for treatment instead trying to diagnose what is causing the damage. The current approach for pain disorders is to take a pill or a potion to cover a symptom instead of getting to the root cause of their disorder. This approach to pain and suffering has to stop!

One popular mind-set for treating pain and inflammation is "Just take anti-inflammatories." It is not that simple, because you might get some relief, but you haven't fixed the problem. That is like saying,

"You know, my sunburned back hurts. Put aloe on it." The aloe might make it feel better and encourage healing, but what good is it doing if you don't come out of the sun? Do you get it? If you have ever had a sunburn, then you have experienced what swollen tissues feel like in the body. Ouch! It hurts.

> **Pain and inflammation! The very things that warn someone damage is occurring and initiate the healing process have also been the target for treatment instead of trying to diagnose what is causing the damage.**

If you have joints that are painful, or you have receptors inflamed around areas like muscles, ligaments, tendons, and joints, they can be extremely painful, like a sunburn. When someone rubs the skin on top of the leg, it should not be painful. If that same leg is placed out in the hot sun about eight hours, it will become red, inflamed, and painful (sunburned). If you rub that same leg that had no pain prior to getting sunburned, it will be extremely sensitive and painful. The skin cells get damaged and the area inflames to initiate healing in that leg. The area becomes painful to warn you so you do not cause further irritation. The body is doing its job to facilitate healing and protect it from further damage. The last thing you want to do is work against the body's natural mechanism of healing. If you can understand a sunburn, you can understand how pain and inflammation work in the body and what they are trying to report. Got it? Let's take it a step further. Consider the possibility of a few million receptors in your body becoming sunburned at the same time. Can you imagine what that might feel like? Patients who have chronic debilitating pain know exactly what it feels like. They often use statements like these to express what they are feeling:

"I don't understand why my whole body hurts."

"It hurts so bad when I get up and move around."

"It hurts when I sit or lie down."

"It hurts when I touch it."

"It hurts even when I don't touch it."

"I ache and feel stiff and sore all over."

"The pain is excruciating and it never lets up."

"It hurts when I turn my head or bend over."

"My back hurts. My joints hurt. My muscles hurt. My head hurts."

Everything Hurts

Yes, you are internally sunburned. You are internally damaged. You are inflamed and that is why you experience pain. Everything becomes more sensitive. Like the sunburned leg, once it is damaged, even the lightest touch can cause a great amount of pain. Is this making sense? That is why the title of this book is "**STOP THE PAIN.**" You have to go to the cause, treat the cause, and the pain will take care of itself. When the rate of repair exceeds the rate of damage, that is the sure sign that the progression of healing is taking place. In order to STOP THE PAIN the focus needs to be on the problem and not the pain.

NF-κB and Nrf2

There are two complexes that work together in the body as a type of check and balance for inflammatory responses, **NF-κB** and **Nrf2**.

NF-kB

NF-κB (nuclear factor kappa-light-chain-enhancer of activated B cells) is a protein complex that controls transcription of DNA, cytokine production, and cell survival. NF-κB is found in almost all animal cell types and is involved in cellular responses to stimuli such as stress, cytokines, free radicals, heavy metals, ultraviolet irradiation, oxidized LDL, and bacterial or viral antigens. NF-κB plays a key role in regulating the immune response to infection. Incorrect regulation of NF-κB has been linked to cancer, inflammatory and autoimmune diseases, septic shock, viral infection, and improper immune development. NF-κB has also been shown to affect memory and the brain's ability to regenerate. NF-κB could be looked at as the "Hulk of inflammation." Every time it shows up something gets damaged.

Nrf2

Nuclear factor (erythroid-derived 2)-like 2, also known as NFE2L2 or Nrf2, is a transcription factor that in humans is encoded by the NFE2L2 gene. Nrf2 is a basic leucine zipper (bZIP) protein that regulates the expression of antioxidant proteins that protect against oxidative damage triggered by injury and inflammation. It activates over 500 genes, most of which are designed to protect the cells, especially by activating anti-oxidation mechanisms in the system. Nrf2 helps to stimulate detoxification and helps the body to get rid of the poisons and pollutants that accumulate in our bodies, like xenobiotics and heavy metals.

Here's an easier way to understand these protein complexes and how they affect inflammatory responses in the system. Let's consider NF-κB to be the "Hulk of inflammation." When left unchallenged in the system it can cause extensive damage to cells and tissues. Who would want the Hulk of inflammation smashing their cells and wrecking their body? When cytokines, oxidation, and free radicals are produced in the system, the very things discussed throughout this book, they make Hulk rage and "HULK SMASH" is the result. Extensive cell damage, systemic inflammation, degeneration, debilitating chronic pain and suffering are the result if left unchallenged.

When the body produces and maintains adequate levels of Nrf2, it's like putting Hulk back in the cage. The damage stops and the body starts to repair the damage. It's far better to live with Hulk inside the cage instead of on the loose causing widespread destruction. Obviously then, the goal is to raise Nrf2 levels and lower the levels of NF-κB. Eating foods such as cruciferous vegetables (broccoli, cauliflower, cabbage, etc.) that are rich in a compound called sulforaphane, activates Nrf2 pathways and improves fat metabolism by improving mitochondrial function.[1] Wow! That's a lot of bang for the buck. Grandma was right when she told you to eat your broccoli, and if you will do what she said, science proves you can lose unwanted body fat and have a lot more energy as a result.

The following foods have been shown to improve the levels of Nrf2 in the body:

Cruciferous vegetables (broccoli, cauliflower, cabbage, brussel sprouts, bok choy) due to their sulforaphane content.
Leafy greens (kale, swiss chard, collard greens, spinach)
Berries (blueberries, raspberries, blackberries)
Olives
Onion
Garlic

Natural compounds that research shows raises Nrf2 levels:

1. Resveratrol

2. Green tea catechins

3. Curcumin

4. Sulforaphane

One popular study showed that eight weeks of consistent prayer and meditation, for at least 15 minutes a day, spread out a couple of times a day, increases Nrf2 activity in the body, which puts Hulk back in his cage by lowering levels of NF-κB. When Hulk is back in his cage, inflammation is reduced. The apostle Paul instructed his followers to pray continually. Wow! He probably had no idea, but he basically told them how to raise Nrf2 levels so Hulk would stop smashing their bodies. It appears there's all kind of healing benefits to be revealed from the Scriptures.

Another excellent way to increase levels of Nrf2 is a technique in exercising called **H.I.I.T. training**. It stands for high intensity interval training. The focus is not as much on the specific types of exercise, but more on the way you perform them. The technique is routinely performed by doing short bursts of basically giving it all you've got while doing the exercise of choice, then backing off to a much slower pace, and continue alternating between the two until the workout is complete. There are literally hundreds of videos on the Internet that demonstrate this technique. If you are going to take the time to exercise, your time is your most precious commodity. Why not get the most bang for your buck, stop wasting time walking around taking breaks throughout the workout. Get in there, do some H.I.I.T. training, work hard, stay consistent, and get out. It should be that simple. This style of training significantly increases

Nrf2 levels, lowers NF-κB by putting Hulk back in his cage, which reduces the levels of inflammation in the body. Studies show that doing H.I.I.T. training for as little as six minutes per day can have a significant impact on improving Nrf2 levels and reducing inflammation in the system. One minute going all out followed by two minutes of a slower pace and continually repeating that cycle for six minutes minimum per day is a pretty small price to pay to get rid of the inflammation in your body. Start today while you are motivated. The hardest part of any training program is getting started and forming a routine. Begin right away before your mind gets involved and starts making excuses on all the reasons why you can't do it. Remember, excuses are nothing more than permission to fail. Start right away, put Hulk back in the cage so you can STOP THE PAIN.

> ❝ Excuses are nothing more than permission to fail. ❞

Brain Pain ("It's all in your head")

Excitotoxins and Microglial Activation

If you have been dealing with depression, forgetfulness, or suffering from migraines, pay close attention. When inflammatory cytokines are released in the body, they activate a process called **microglial activation.** You do not have to know all these terms, but make sure you get the gist of what is being explained. The microglia are **macrophages**. A macrophage is a scavenger cell. Did you ever play the game, Pac-Man? Once the game got started you would see the little yellow round guy eat the pellets as he said, "Waka, waka, waka, waka, waka, waka, waka, waka, waka, waka." That is what a macrophage does in your body. It goes around, gobbles up the bad cells and debris. The macrophages in your liver are called Kupffer cells, monocytes in the blood, histocytes in the skin, etc.. The ones in your brain are microglial cells.

Once you have initiated the Pac-Man in the brain, they start to clean up the debris, "Waka, waka, waka, waka, waka, waka." And every time they eat, they release a molecule called glutamate. Once it is released, glutamate stimulates what is called a NMDA receptor; the NMDA receptor then releases calcium into the brain cell (neuron) and excites that cell to death.

Substances that provoke this process are called excitotoxins because they cause microglial activation that excites the nerve cells to death. Excitotoxins are substances like the artificial sweetener aspartame, or the food flavor enhancer monosodium glutamate (MSG). I can tell you from personal experience that either one of those excititoxins practically wreck my system if I consume them. They cause almost immediate burning and aching pain in my neck, upper back, and shoulders. Yes, excititoxins can produce pain in your body as well as a host of other symptoms. The pain can last for several days until the system clears the toxins. Studies have shown promising results that **pregnenolone** can actually stop the microglial activation caused from these excititoxins. Pregnenolone is a steroid hormone that is directly produced by the brain, which is why it is defined as a **neurosteroid**. Pregnenolone carries out several cerebral functions, such as neuroprotection, neuroplasticity, and neurogenesis; moreover, it regulates the mood and the memory.[2] This simply means it protects, repairs, and regenerates the brain and the nervous system, while also dictating what your mood will be and what you will and won't remember. That's a pretty big deal. If you've been using MSG or aspartame, perhaps it would be a good idea to stop consuming them and start taking some pregnenolone. Do we really want prolonged microglial activation in the brain? If microglial activation is happening in the brain, neurons are being damaged. When there is damage, what comes next? Inflammation. The inflammation produces pain and soreness and the cycle of pain is initiated once again. Once this vicious inflammatory cycle starts in the brain it can cause unexplained headaches that usually get misdiagnosed. If you have headaches and have tried everything to relieve them with no success, this may be one scenario to consider. If the problem is left untreated for 20 to 30 years, it can cause chronic brain inflammation, degeneration, and finally progress into Alzheimer's, which is a form of dementia. Alzheimer's is a 20-30 year process. It is caused from chronic brain inflammation that leads to chronic degeneration. When you look at pictures of a brain, it looks like a bunch of mountains and valleys. When those mountains get lower and the valleys get wider, that is the classic sign of brain degeneration caused from chronic inflammation. One of the causes of this can be prolonged microglial activation. Think about it, how well does anything work if it swells?

Have you ever had a swollen arm or a swollen finger? Have you ever jammed your finger? If so, were you able to do the tasks that you wanted to do as easily and efficiently as before you injured it? A swollen finger can even get to the point where you can't bend it. With this in mind, does inflammation help function or generally hinder it? If this is the case with the finger, you can imagine what inflammation can do in other more sensitive parts of your body.

Why is that important? Well, we were just talking about the brain. Most everyone likes to have good focus, don't they? They like to have a good memory with total recall. Well, what would happen if brain function were impaired? Do you suppose some of the focus and function might change?

If you've ever had **brain fog**, then you most likely also had some sort of immune activation or microglial activation that created inflammation in your brain. The cell damage created from the inflammation most likely caused some brain dysfunction, which affected the thought process, which, in turn, caused unclear thinking—better known as brain fog.

A good friend of mine, and a former Miss America, started having severe memory problems and was even starting to struggle remembering her parts while playing the piano. She is an accomplished pianist and an extremely gifted singer, songwriter, and musician. You can imagine how frustrating it might be when the very thing you are called to do in life becomes threatened by health complications. After becoming educated on aspartame (NutraSweet, an artificial sweetener that is an excitotoxin) and how it can cause toxic effects that damage and even destroy brain cells, she stopped drinking diet drinks. A few months later she fully regained her memory as well as her ability to remember and play her music.

I have often wondered what might have happened if she continued consuming the aspartame. Would the process have continued until it finally reached critical mass causing her to be debilitated? It appears to be one of those "things that make you go 'Hmmmmm!'"

Alzheimer's and Dementia

Science has proven that the majority of the cases of depression are caused from brain inflammation. An inflamed brain can affect neural pathways and other related parts of the brain that keep the mood balanced. When inflammation starts from brain cells being damaged, the gating mechanisms begin to fail. This, in turn, causes neurological changes that down regulate the neurotransmitters. What does all that mean? When our bodies encounter substances or trauma that damage cells causing inflammation, depression is commonly seen as a result of the insult. These processes serve as neuro-logical disrupters and can have devastating effects on your health.

Many doctors are not informed of the newer science and still embrace treatment protocols that, in most cases, bring short-term benefit or no benefit at all. Due to the new research, it seems quite obvious that the focus of treatment for depression should be at-tempting to find the cause of the inflammation and develop strat-egies to prevent it. However, it is common practice to, instead, put someone on a drug as a way to enhance the neurotransmitter. Why not work on the brain inflammation instead?

How much have you heard in the media lately about dementia? Alzheimer's? Did you know that these degenerative brain condi-tions are some of the fastest diseases on the rise? Research clearly shows they are a twenty to thirty, to even a forty-year disease. It starts around the age of the thirty and forty year olds, and the brain starts to inflame. This is about the same time frame most people that deal with unexplained depression start to become depressed. After twenty or thirty years of this, when studying the effects on the anatomy of the human brain, one of the first things you notice is that the hills and valleys become affected. Have you ever seen a brain? Have you seen pictures of the brain? When those hills start getting shorter and the valleys start getting wider, that means the brain is degenerating.

I am trying to get your attention and I hope it is working because if you leave suppressed inflammation, pressure, deactivation, and the glutamate response, prolonged, the brain continues to degenerate.

Next it initiates the formation of neurofibrillary tangles which in turn starts the process of phosphorylation of proteins, which simply means how you turn a protein on or off. This leads to clumping in the brain; and the brain neurofibrillary tangles start to tangle with that clumping. These clumps and tangles are called **beta-amyloid plaques**. You might as well learn that term now because you are probably going to be seeing it in magazines and on the news for years to come. When these beta-amyloid plaques accumulate in high quantity, they are a classic sign that dementia is getting worse in the brain. Alzheimer's is a form of dementia. All dementia is not Alzheimer's. All Alzheimer's is dementia. When the demented brain or the degenerative brain gets older these plaques continue to form until finally function is impaired. The worse the plaques, the worse the dementia. The scientific community is still debating whether the plaque is the problem, or as the more current research reveals, instead it's a patching mechanism that's the evidence that the body is trying to heal the damaged areas. Either way they get progressively worse as the brain continues to degenerate. The longer it stays inflamed, the more symptoms will be displayed. It starts in a subtle fashion. Someone may walk into a room and cannot remember why they are there. They see someone; they know them, but they cannot recall their name. The other parts of their brain seem to be intact yet as it slowly progresses, things start to get worse. Eventually as everything gets worse, it can get to the place where they cannot discern anyone or anything in their life, and they walk around helpless, and live in their own world — all because someone did not explain to them this information so they would know how to stop the inflammation that caused it. If you can stop the inflammation now, in twenty or thirty years you will not have to worry about having this horrible disease.

Neurotransmitters in Gut

Remember, most of the neurotransmitters used by the brain are made in the gut and are what assists your brain in maintaining its balance so it can efficiently run the body. Four of the predominant neurotransmitters used in the brain that balance our mental state are: **serotonin** that improves our moods and enhances the sense of well-being, **dopamine** that motivates us and gives us drive, **norepinephrine** that mobilizes the body and gets it ready for action, and **GABA** that helps us to relax and be able to sleep at night. These explanations are basic examples of neurotransmitter function and are certainly more complex in their influence in the body. These particular brain chemicals work to keep our systems from revving up or slowing down and help us to stay balanced.

If they ever become imbalanced, they can upset the balance of a lot of the other hormones in the body as well. The brain chemicals are mostly made in the gut. If the gut has an immune activation and it causes the gut to inflame, the same way inflammation affected the finger so it could not function properly, the gut function can also be impaired affecting its function as well. That dysfunction can most certainly affect the production of neurotransmitters being produced by the gut, creating a shortage. This shortage can dramatically affect the brain's ability to stabilize the mood, causing a severe imbalance in brain chemistry as well as the body's physiology. Certain foods, chemicals, substances, and toxins can severely disrupt this delicate balance as well. The occurrence of this severe imbalance and its effect on brain balance is what drives so many people to ask the question, "Why do I feel so depressed?" Instead of trying to understand this process and try to correct it, those who suffer from this disorder join so many others who are prescribed a pill for their depression that usually only gives temporary relief, if any, while the underlying problem is left untreated. This allows it to progress causing further imbalance and the vicious cycle continues once again. Depression is a complicated disorder and recommending a pill to try to make the uptake of a neurotransmitter continue to hold the system intact may be a necessary Band-Aid, but the root cause has to be addressed if the patient is ever going to fully recover. I am all for the use of medications as long as they are used as a crutch in conjunction with a combined strategy that focuses on treating the real problem until they can stand on their own.

What I do not approve of is when medication is prescribed for people in order to pacify them, instead of doing what is required to find the root of the problem. The sad truth is doctors often tell people that the problems they are having are all in their head. That's a polite way of saying, "We can't find anything wrong so you must be the problem." In many of those cases the problem is not in their head, it's in their gut. Once again, keep in mind that most of the neuro-chemicals used in your brain are actually manufactured in your gut. They are processed by the brain. If the gut is messed up, every-thing is messed up. People who suffer from unexplained depression should always consider the gut as at least part of or perhaps the root of the problem. In some cases it might be as simple as **fix the gut = fix the brain**.

Leaky Gut = Leaky Brain

The gastrointestinal tract consists of an enormous surface area. Its entire surface area measurement totals up to about 400 square yards. That's equivalent to the surface area of about two tennis courts. It has to maintain a tight barrier against the ingress of harmful substances, keeping the good guys in and the bad guys out. There are many things that cause the breakdown of this crucial barrier over time. This barrier must be preserved in order to stay healthy. Disruption of this barrier results in what's referred to as **"increased intestinal permeability."** That means the barrier starts to leak. This allows things to leak out into the system. The medical term for this condition is called **"leaky gut syndrome."** When this occurs it allows harmful substances and pathogens to pass into the bloodstream. This initiates a systemic immune activation and the entire vicious inflammatory cycle repeats itself. When poor gut health, an imbalanced microbiome, and a poor diet are present, the barrier suffers damage causing it to leak. When this barrier leaks it causes systemic issues that cause other barriers to leak as well. One important structure that's damaged and affected by this process is the **blood brain barrier**. When this barrier is breached it is referred to as "**leaky brain syndrome**." This can cause brain inflammation which produces disorders like depression, anxiety, pain syndromes, headaches, and brain fog. Yes, the gut affects the brain and the brain affects the body. The brain can cause the pain, "**Brain Pain!**" When the gut barrier leaks and releases toxins into the system it stimulates pro-inflammatory cytokines that can inflame the brain and disrupt the endocrine balance, and as a result, the thyroid gland is often affected hindering its function. One of the first symptoms of an underactive thyroid is a sluggish digestive system. Lack of thyroid function directly affects gut assimilation and absorption. Can you see this started in the gut and has now cycled back and is affecting the gut? This creates a vicious destructive cycle that keeps branching out, affecting more and more systems until finally the entire body suffers damage from this devastating process. The cycle looks like this:

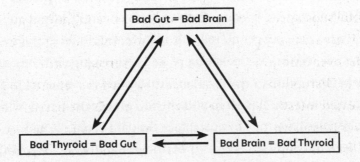

This is one of the most common yet frustrating cycles to be stuck in. Over time this cycle of events can really take its toll on someone's health. The problem is when someone is suffering from this condition there are no routine lab tests for diagnosing leaky gut. There's none for leaky brain either. Routine TSH and T4 testing for thyroid returns normal on plenty of people who have a subclinical hypothyroid condition so it usually goes undetected as well. The patient goes to their physician and gets these routine exam and lab tests. The exam returns normal, the blood levels look great, but the person still feels terrible. They get sent home with no diagnosis and no hope for recovery. When each organ involved is deficient, it produces a patient profile that's specific to its dysfunction.

Here's a depiction of what the typical profiles look like in chart form:

Thyroid (Fat, Fatigued, Female)

Brain (Stressed, Suppressed, Sleepless)

Gut (Constipated, Complicated, Chronic)

Of course these are generalities and the symptom profiles may vary. For example, a male may certainly also have a thyroid problem, etc. Fixing these problems requires correcting all of the other issues previously discussed that ultimately wind up culminating in the brain. I personally know of many patients who have had these chronic problems and pain for years. They've been referred from specialist to specialist, yet still get no relief or resolve. Could it be that everyone was looking in the wrong place? If you happen to be one of those patients whose condition has frustrated your doctors to the point they tell you, "It's all in your head," give them a copy of this book because they may be correct. Brain pain is real. It may be all in your head but you are certainly not imagining it. FIX THE SIX and follow the recommendations in this book so you can be educated on how to STOP THE PAIN in your brain.

Epigenetics

The word **genetics** is a universal term. The term basically refers to the chromosomal patterns and pairs that you get from your parents and descendants that makes you, you. There is another term, **genotype**, that refers to the probability of a gene expressing itself within an individual. An example of this would be, if my grandmother had heart disease and my father had heart disease, I am probably going to have heart disease because it is in my genotype. That is not an absolute and does not mean I am going to; it means I have a higher probability, thus the term genotype.

If my genotype is heart disease that doesn't mean it will automatically manifest in my body. It doesn't mean I will also have heart disease one day. It does refer to the fact that there's a higher probability of contracting heart disease if I make poor choices and don't do the right things to prevent it. When we abuse our bodies this way, the genes mutate and express themselves, and just like Grandma and Father, the heart genotype expresses itself and heart disease is the result. Once this occurs the genotype becomes the **phenotype**. What is truly interesting

> **❝...you don't have to just accept the family genetic curses being handed down to you. Do things to prevent them instead of just sitting around hoping you don't get them.❞**

is just because you have something in your gene pool does not mean that you will necessarily express it in your lifetime. That means if you are placed in the wrong set of circumstances under wrong conditions, then that inherited disease producing potential would be able to express itself and you would contract that disease; whereas if you could be placed in the right environment under the right set of conditions, there would be no reason for the inherited disease producing potential to ever express itself. That's why some individuals have diseases in their family history, yet they never wind up with any of those diseases. Their genetic potentials have not been stressed by the factors and conditions that cause these diseases to manifest. What does all that mean? It means you don't have to just accept the family genetic curses being handed down to you. Do things to prevent them instead of just sitting around hoping you don't get them.

There is a whole field of study called **epigenetics**. What is an epigenetic? It's the study of changes in organisms caused by modification of gene expression rather than alteration of the genetic code itself. A very basic definition would be, the study of biological mechanisms that will switch genes on and off. This field of study has transformed the way we think about genomes. It's all about how genes are expressed and used, rather than the DNA sequence of the genes themselves. We know a part of how epigenetics work is by adding and removing small chemical tags to DNA. You might want to think of these chemical tags as master keys that connect to particular genes with information about whether they should be switched on or off. DNA from humans is made up of approximately 3 billion nucleotide bases. There are four fundamental types of bases that comprise DNA (adenine, cytosine, guanine, and thymine commonly abbreviated as A, C, G, and T). These chemical tags, or master keys, are called methyl groups and are used to modify one of these four bases. The sequence of the bases is what determines the order of the building blocks that construct our lives. Genes are specific sequences of bases that provide instructions on how to make important proteins that trigger various biological actions to carry out life functions. Epigenetics control genes by either turning them on or turning them off. Stresses of every kind, to include but not limited to environmental, electromagnetic, chemical, physical, temperature, trauma, all influence the genes in how they express.

When the genes are under the wrong conditions they may become stressed to the point where the master key switches on one of the bad expressions such as an **oncogene** (a cancer causing gene). That person's epigenetics will initiate that new genetic expression and start producing cancer cells in that body. Depending on what is switched on or off determines what will and what will not be expressed. That explains why people can be perfectly healthy their entire life until they have a traumatic experience. The genes get stressed, they switch on a bad expression, and they find themselves dealing with a disease or disorder soon thereafter. I had a patient come to my office who had a severe autoimmune disease called Sjögren's syndrome. She was already in the advanced stages and was going over the history of the onset of her disease. She explained to me that she had been a normal person, leading a normal life, always had lots of energy, and considered herself to be ridiculously healthy. She was involved in a head-on collision in her vehicle and sustained some pretty nasty injuries. She told me that from that day forward she began to experience a shift in her system. From that day the disease manifested and progressively continued to get worse. The disease had advanced so far by the time she reached my office, that all I could offer was palliative care. A couple of years later she passed away from the effects of the disease. The doctors all agreed that the trauma from the accident caused that genetic predisposition to express itself.

Sometimes things happen in life that are completely out of our control However, I've also had patients who have had genetic conditions that they overcame insurmountable odds and have had success leading normal lives.

That reminds me of another patient of mine who I treated almost thirty years ago, who had a rare disease called tublerosclerosis. She was a young girl about the age of six whose feet were turning in. The mother wanted to know if I could help. During the history the mother told me that her daughter wasn't expected to live past the age of eleven or twelve because that was the prognosis for that disease. She also reported that because of all of the tumors in her brain that she was having seizures throughout the majority of the day. That was apparently common for that stage of the disease.

I agreed to help her with the feet issue but I also asked her if she minded if I treated her to see if I could reduce the seizure activity. After finishing the exam and reviewing her x-rays, I decided on a treatment protocol that I felt would provide her with the best results. After the first treatment she never had another seizure. Prior to coming to my office she was almost despondent and had very little social interaction. After she completed all of her treatments she was very outgoing and was an extremely pleasant child. I actually feel tears welling up in my eyes writing about it. She finally moved away but a few years ago I happened to run into her mother who told me she was still living a fulfilled life and was just as outgoing and pleasant as she had been with no regression from the disease. The moral of the story is, genes can be switched on and they also can be switched off. The good news is we do have some control over this occurrence. When we make our bodies healthy by making the right choices and

❝...health is a choice, choose life.❞

doing the right things consistently, we make the system much more resistant to the stresses caused from our external world. Following good advice like the instruction in this book can have a significant impact on how and what your epigenetics will be expressing in the future. Just as the bad gene expressions were switched on by doing wrong things, they can certainly be switched back off from doing the right things. Sometimes "health is a choice, choose life."

Methylation MTHFR

There is a process in the body called **methylation**. Methylation involves the conversion of a simple amino acid **methionine**. If the correct nutrients are present it is converted to **homocysteine** and finally to **glutathione**. This conversion is necessary because glutathione is the "**master antioxidant**" in the body. If its conversion is not completed properly, the results will be elevated homocysteine levels. Homocysteine is an extremely inflammatory by-product. Excess levels can produce all kinds of damaging inflammatory effects in the body, especially in the vascular system. The reason is because homocysteine produces molecules that cause inflammation and also causes oxidation in the system. When it's properly converted to glutathione, it becomes the master antioxidant in the body and actually works to reduce inflammation. Therefore, this conversion is vital for good health.

Glutathione is comprised of three amino acids **glutamine**, **glycine**, and **cysteine**. It also contains a sulfur compound as part of its make-up that makes it extremely powerful. Depending on the source that you are quoting, it's anywhere in the concentration of a hundred to a thousand times stronger than vitamin C in antioxidant capability. Glutathione levels have to be preserved in the body or survival wouldn't be possible. If it's not, so much damage would be caused it would be hard to ever recover. A good example of this is when someone drinks alcohol excessively (more than 3 drinks daily) and then takes a high dose of acetaminophen over several doses. This scenario can dramatically drop the levels of glutathione in the system to a critical status and many people die as a result.[3] When people have impaired methylation that cause lowered glutathione levels, they usually wind up with inflammatory degenerative disorders. One of the first symptoms people have with glutathione deficiency is pain. It's usually systemic pain and can be one of the primary causes of disorders such as fibromyalgia, chronic fatigue syndrome, inflammatory arthritis, migraines, and a host of other problems that produce significant pain. Optimal glutathione levels are necessary to maintain the integrity of the system. Maintaining these levels is essential for the treatment and prevention of chronic pain.

The methylation process also is responsible for the conversions necessary to produce a substance called **SAMe**. SAM-e is a nutrient that helps balance and regulate the neurotransmitters in the brain, especially for those who are prone to experience symptoms of depression.

If homocysteine levels are elevated, the probability of getting Alzheimer's doubles. It doubles your chances of developing inflammatory heart conditions, arterial sclerosis, atherosclerosis, and even osteoporosis. The higher it is elevated, you just keep doubling the risk. Some studies show the risk of heart attacks elevate to ten times the likelihood with moderate elevations in homocysteine. Depending on how high it's elevated, the reality of it continues to exponentially increase your odds of inflammatory destruction that ultimately wind up causing a potentially life-threatening disease.

The good news is that with the addition of only 4 nutrients into the diet, the homocysteine levels can usually be lowered within a few weeks.

The four nutrients are:

1. B12 (preferably methylcobalamine) 1,000 mcg.

2. B6 15-25 mg.

3. Folate (in the converted form methyltetrahydrafolate) dose dependent

4. N-acetyl cysteine (NAC) is the precursor of glutathione 3,000 mg.

If these nutrients are present and the gut is not too inflamed to absorb them, the system should be enabled to make the necessary conversions and the balance of homocysteine, glutathione, and SAMe should improve. However, in some cases, especially chronic ones, supplementing with SAMe and/or glutathione (liposomal or IV) may be necessary.

Natural Medicine to the Rescue

STOP THE PAIN PROTOCOLS:

I have discussed in detail the benefits of multiple natural compounds, nutrients, plant extracts, neutraceuticals, minerals, antioxidants, and cofactors. Sometimes it's difficult to figure out how to put them all together in order to maximize their effectiveness. Over the past three decades I have assembled nutrient protocols of these natural substances that directly address the problems discussed in this book. Choose the protocol that applies to your situation, or relates to the health issue you are dealing with. If you choose more than one category, that's okay, the protocols can be combined. They are listed in order of the steps to recover. This is designed for those who want to recover all of the systems listed in the **SIX TO FIX**

RECOVERY SYSTEM. The strategy is to follow each protocol one at a time for thirty days each until all six are completed. For those who have more damage in one area than another may need to continue doing that protocol in combination with the others as you complete the six month Six to Fix Recovery System.

The gut is a good example of this. The gut usually takes three months minimum to fully recover in people who have significant gut issues. To invest six months time to repair years of damage, as well as provide protection for the future, seems pretty reasonable.

> **There are two things that motivate people, inspiration and desperation.**

The best plan when taking multiple packs is to spread them out throughout the day. For example, you may take a pack of ADRENAL SUPPORT combined with three or four MEGA EPAs with your breakfast meal. At lunch you may combine INFLA-IMMUNE and MI-TOGEN and take together with the meal. You may take LIPOGEST and three or four INCELLATE with the evening meal and perhaps take INFLA-OX and INFLA-OIL about an hour or two before bedtime. Actually that's my personal nutrient regimen that I take daily as well as taking three to five CELLZYME with meals to help with good digestion, DAILY ESSENTIALS taken every other day, and BM SUPPORT either upon wakening or right at bedtime. I do practice what I preach and am a living testimony of the results this information can provide. My best testimony in life is "I am the happiest, healthiest, most energetic person I know." Sometimes I actually get on my own nerves.

There are two things that motivate people, inspiration and desperation. My greatest hope is that you'll choose to get inspired to do something now, so you aren't forced to do something out of desperation later.

Six to Fix Recovery Protocols:

1) Inflammation and Oxidation Recovery Protocol:

a) **INFLA-OX** – contains resveratrol, green tea catechins and other natural ingredients that research has shown to reduce the effects of oxidation and inflammation by improving Nrf2 levels and reducing NFkb levels. (Take one pack with a meal.)

b) **INFLA-IMMUNE** – contains pine bark and grape seed extract along with other antioxidants, neutraceuticals, and natural ingredients that research suggests helps to improve the process of tissue regeneration, repair, and improving healing time in damaged or injured tissues. Research also suggests they reduce and improve oxidation and inflammation that can reduce pain and improve immune function. (Take one pack with a meal.)

c) **INFLA-OILS** – Contains 3 oils that research has shown to be beneficial in reducing and improving inflammation in the joints and in the body. They've also been shown to enhance the immune system and improve the body's defense system. (Take one pack with a meal.)

d) **MEGA EPA** – contains concentrated fish oils that research has shown to reduce inflammation and relieve pain and discomfort. The body, for proper repair and lubrication, needs essential fatty acids. Normal joint linings are well lubricated and structurally intact and therefore should not be painful. When joints get damaged and or lose proper lubrication, the results can be debilitating pain and discomfort. (Take two to three capsules with a meal.)

2) Gut Recovery Protocol:

a) **COLO-CLEANSE** – contains nutrients and compounds research has shown improve the digestive system. Insoluble fiber that works as a bulking agent to pull water into bowel to make stool a soft consistency to avoid straining which can help prevent hemorrhoids, diverticula, and/or aneurysms. Flax seed that coats and lubricates the bowel which helps transit time to prevent waste products from being held against colon wall. Alfalfa that assists cleansing the colon and helps to remove the toxins that can provoke allergies and sensitivities. Caprylic acid to help prevent overgrowth of yeast and bad bacteria. Grapefruit seed extract that has antimicrobial activity. Fructooligosaccharides to promote growth of the good bacteria. Spanish black radish to assist in cleansing upper G.I. tract and to help increase secretion and also stimulates digestive enzymes to assist in absorbing of nutrients. Aloe Vera to help to soothe and promote healing throughout the complete digestive tract. Mg-B12 that helps to rid toxins (metals, chemicals, etc.) from the body. (One pack a.m. – one pack p.m.)

b) **BIOCLEANSE** – contains natural compounds that research shows can rid intestinal parasites, unwanted yeast, and bad bugs. It also repopulates the gut with the good intestinal flora, which are referred to as probiotics, assisting in restoring the microbiome back to a normal state of balance. (One pack a.m. - one pack p.m.)

c) **L-GLUTAMINE** – is the amino acid the body uses to repair the endothelial linings in the gut and in the body. Current research suggests that higher doses of 25-30 grams daily for three to six months are usually required in order to restore the linings back to normal.

d) **MINSORB** – contains highly absorbable minerals that research has shown to be beneficial for normal growth, repair, and function in the body. Minerals are utilized by the body for anything from healing and repair to detoxification, bowel function, energy production, and mobility/flexibility/agility. (Two to four capsules daily with a meal.)

e) **BM SUPPORT** – provides ground psyllium husk capsules that are an insoluble fiber that works as a bulking agent to pull water into bowel to make stool a soft consistency. (Eight to ten capsules upon awakening or at bedtime with 12 or more ounces of water.)

f) **PROBIOTICS** – contain several strains of normal gut flora that research shows are necessary for normal gut function. They assist the body in restoring, balancing, and maintaining the gut microbiome. (Take one capsule daily with a meal.)

3) JOINT RECOVERY PROTOCOL:

a) **JOINT COMPOUND** – contains ingredients that research shows may help relieve joint pain, swelling, and discomfort. When joint linings become inflamed from degenerative processes, they need the right nutrients in order to be repaired properly. When the linings are healed, things like inflammation, pain, soreness and stiffness in these previously damaged areas should all normalize as a result. (One to two packs daily.)

b) **COLLAGEN PROTEIN** – contains ingredients that research shows may assist in the repair and regeneration of collagen tissues. Joint linings, tissues that support the human frame, and the cells in skin, hair, and nails, all have collagen fibers that need repaired to stay youthful and healthy. It also has an excellent array of amino acids. Amino acids are the building blocks in nature that rebuild and repair our systems. Maintaining adequate levels are necessary for optimal healing and repair for the body. Sometimes when muscles and joints become sore, stiff, and inflamed is because the tissues are damaging faster than they are repairing. This can occur from exercise, traumas, or even overdoing it while working in the yard. Individuals who have been suffering from chronic pain and/or sickness can also be plagued with this problem. Providing amino acids in the diet helps to optimize the potential to repair so the tissues can heal and recover from the damage. (Mix 30 - 40 grams in eight to ten ounces of water.)

c) **INFLA-OILS** – Contains three oils that research has shown to be beneficial in reducing and improving inflammation in the joints and in the body. They've also been shown to enhance the immune system and improve the body's defense system. (Take one pack with a meal.)

d) **PAIN-X** – contains natural compounds that research has shown to be beneficial in relieving pain and discomfort without the harmful side effect that can be experienced from taking non-steroidal anti-inflammatory drugs. These compounds are not addictive and can be used for long periods of time if well tolerated. (Take two to four capsules with food as needed for relief.)

e) **MEGA EPA** – contains concentrated fish oils that research has shown to reduce inflammation and relieve pain and discomfort. Essential fatty acids are needed by the body for proper repair and lubrication. Normal joint linings are well lubricated and structurally intact and therefore should not be painful. When joints get damaged and/or lose proper lubrication, the results can be debilitating pain and discomfort. (Take two to three capsules one time daily; depending on severity of condition more may be necessary.)

f) **MINSORB** – contains highly absorbable minerals that research has shown to be beneficial for normal growth, repair, and function in the body. Minerals are utilized by the body for anything from healing and repair to detoxification, bowel function, energy production, and mobility/flexibility/agility. (Take two to four capsules daily.)

4) Mitochondrial (Energy) Recovery Protocol:

a) **ADRENAL SUPPORT** – contains nutrients, natural compounds, and neutraceuticals, that research has shown to assist the body in recovering from the harmful effects of stress. There are millions of people who suffer from the devastating effects that intense stress can cause in their bodies. Trauma, mechanical, physical, chemical, pain, emotional stresses etc., can all wreak havoc on the body. Prolonged stresses, can weaken the adrenal system and lower the body's ability to be able to heal and recover normally. These stresses can create significant deficiencies that not only prevent the body from repairing properly, but can also add to the problem making it even worse. Fatigue and exhaustion are common in individuals who suffer from adrenal insufficiency. Adrenal recovery is essential in anyone who is trying to recover from pain and suffering especially when stress has been associated with the cause. (Take one pack with breakfast - one pack with lunch.) Note: if doing intermittent fasting, eliminate the morning dose.

b) **ALA/ALC** – research suggests that Alpha Lipoic Acid is a powerful antioxidant made inside of the mitochondria that converts nutrients into energy, reduces inflammation, improves insulin resistance, slows skin aging, helps stop muscle cramps, and improves nerve function. It also shows that Acetyl-LCarnitine (ALCAR) is a biomarker for depression, primary amino acid involved in burning fats for fuel, crosses blood brain barrier to assist in healthy brain function, significant in forming neurotransmitters in brain to improve function and cognition. (Take 1 capsule with morning meal – one capsule with evening meal.)

c) **MITOGEN** – contains CoQ10 in both the converted and non-converted forms along with other natural ingredients in which research suggests improves mitochondrial function as well as promotes better heart and muscle function. (Take one pack with a meal.)

d) **MINSORB** – contains highly absorbable minerals that research has shown to be beneficial for normal growth, repair, and function in the body. Minerals are utilized by the body for anything from healing and repair to detoxification, bowel function, energy production, and mobility/flexibility/agility. (Take two to four capsules with meals.)

5) Metabolic Recovery Protocol:

a) **LIPOGEST** – contains natural compounds that research has shown assists in the digestion and assimilation of fats. Proper fat metabolism is crucial for maintaining optimal health. Every cell lining in the body has a component of fat in its bi-layer phospholipid membrane. Normal fatty acid metabolism and proper fat assimilation are necessary in order to repair those linings. The by-products of digested fats are also used to lubricate the joint linings and help to prevent them from inflaming and becoming sore and painful. (One pack taken with largest meal of the day.)

b) **TAKE IT OFF** – contains a special blend of amino acids that research has shown to increase the release of Growth Hormone (GH). GH is sometimes referred to as the master regulator of muscle growth. It stimulates cellular reproduction and regeneration. It also regulates carbohydrates and fat metabolism. (Must be taken at bedtime with no food for three hours prior.)

c) **KETOX** – is a group of ketone mineral salts that research suggests provides the body with an alternate source of energy while at the same time provides beneficial minerals that are necessary for adequate recovery from physical exertion and stress. They are excellent for those who need a boost to the metabolism and are stuck and can't lose weight. They are especially helpful when someone is on the keto diet and eats too many carbs, they can immediatly put them back in ketosis without waiting the two or three days it usually takes. These are especially effective while the body's mitochondrial system is initially recovering from chronic damage and disease. Muscle aches, pain, and soreness can be prevalent during periods when the mitochondria and metabolism are functioning poorly. These ketone mineral salts can help to rejuvenate the muscles and alleviate the pain and discomfort.

d) **DAILY ESSENTIALS** – contain vitamins, minerals, cofactors, essential fatty acid, and enzymes that research has shown to assist with normal metabolism and function. They are designed to support the system long term and provide the body with a wide array of nutrients in order to prevent deficiency. (Take one pack daily with a meal.)

e) **Thyroid support** – contains nutrients, natural compounds, herbals, and the amino acid tyrosine which research has shown to assist the thyroid in its normal function. This should only be taken if someone has three or more of the symptoms in the thyroid survey. (Take two capsules three times daily.)

Other Alternatives

1. **Stem cell** – Your own stem cells have the potential to regenerate all kinds of cells of the body. Scientists have developed the technology to differentiate stem cells into neural cell, blood cells, skin cells, and hair cells. These cells may be used to replace the old cells of the body with new and young cells to treat the aging related diseases. I have personally witnessed some pretty impressive results from people recovering from severe debilitating pain syndromes and neurodegenerative conditions by them utilizing stem cell injection therapy. Stem cells detect cytokine signals released by damaged cells and travel to those areas to initiate the healing process. The Department of Health and Human Resources classifies stem cell therapy under the category of **regenerative medicine** and proclaims it as "the next evolution in medical treatments." Stem cell therapies may offer the potential to treat diseases or conditions for which few treatments exist. Sometimes called the body's "master cells," stem cells are the cells that develop into blood, brain, bones, and all of the body's organs. They have the potential to repair, restore, replace, and regenerate cells, and could possibly be used to treat many medical conditions and diseases. Some unscrupulous providers offer stem cell products that are both unapproved and unproven. So beware of potentially dangerous procedures and confirm what's really being offered before you consider any treatment.

2. **Platelet Rich Plasma (PRP) Injections** – Although blood is mainly a liquid (called plasma), it also contains small solid components (red cells, white cells, and platelets). The platelets are best known for their importance in clotting blood. However, platelets also contain

hundreds of proteins called growth factors that are very important in the healing of injuries. PRP is plasma with many more platelets than what is typically found in blood. The concentration of platelets — and, thereby, the concentration of growth factors — can be five to ten times greater (or richer) than usual. To develop a PRP preparation, blood must first be drawn from a patient. The platelets are separated from other blood cells and their concentration is increased during a process called centrifugation. Then the increased concentration of platelets is combined with the remaining blood. PRP can then be carefully injected into the injured area to initiate the healing process. Although it is not exactly clear how PRP works, laboratory studies have shown that the increased concentration of growth factors in PRP can potentially speed up the healing process. Typically, PRP treatments are far less expensive than stem cell and for most are more accessible. This can be an excellent way to overcome traumatic injuries as well as chronic joint pains, especially for those who have not responded to traditional therapies.

3. **Medical Ozone treatments** – Ozone (O_3) gas discovered in the mid-nineteenth century is a molecule consisting of three atoms of oxygen in a dynamically unstable structure due to the presence of mesomeric states. Although O_3 has dangerous effects, researchers believe it has many therapeutic effects. Ozone therapy has been utilized and heavily studied for more than a century. Its effects are proven, consistent, safe, and with minimal and preventable side effects. Medical O_3 is used to disinfect and treat disease. Mechanism of actions is by inactivation of bacteria, viruses, fungi, yeast, and protozoa, stimulation of oxygen metabolism, activation of the immune system.[4] Ozone can be administered by **injection, ultraviolet blood irridation (UBI)** using IV therapy, **rectal insufflation** (basically an ozone gas enema), and even using ozonated oils and drinking ozanated water. These treatments are typically safe and

effective when performed by trained and licensed professionals. Using nasal rinses with freshly ozonated water can be an excellent and efficient way to rid the sinuses of excess microbial overgrowth. However, ozone should never be inhaled, as it is a strong irritant to the lungs. If ozone inhalation occurs the effects can usually be reversed by immediately taking a couple of grams of vitamin C. It is used to treat a host of pain syndromes and usually provides immediate results in some cases. It has been shown to be quite beneficial in the treatment of allergies and sensitivities using both UBI and rectal insufflation. I am a huge fan of ozone and have personally witnessed its powerful healing effects. Sometimes it works so well it seems almost magical. I have personally used it to knock out infections in my own body. It can also be very effective when it's injected along the spine and even the exremities to bring immediate relief of pain from injury to the tendons, muscles, ligaments, and even the myofascia. Drinking freshly ozonated water can also bring a speedy recovery from stomach viruses or flu. The applications are endless with this amazing gas.

4. **Acupuncture** – Acupuncture is a system of integrative medicine that involves pricking the skin or tissues with needles, used to alleviate pain and to treat various physical, mental, and emotional conditions. Originating in ancient China, acupuncture is now widely practiced in the West. Over the years there has been substantial debate about whether acupuncture really works for chronic pain. Research from an international team of experts adds to the evidence that it does provide real relief from common forms of pain. The team pooled the results of 29 studies involving nearly 18,000 participants. Some had acupuncture, some had "sham" acupuncture, and some didn't have acupuncture at all. Overall, acupuncture relieved pain by about 50 percent. The results were published in *Archives of Internal Medicine*.[5]

5. **Homeopathy** – Homeopathy is a system of alternative medicine created in 1796 by Samuel Hahnemann, based on his doctrine of like cures like (similia similibus curentur), a claim that a substance that causes the symptoms of a disease in healthy people would cure similar symptoms in sick people.[6] Homeopathic products come from plants (such as red onion, arnica [mountain herb], poison ivy, belladonna [deadly nightshade], and stinging nettle), minerals (such as white arsenic), or animals (such as crushed whole bees). Homeopathic products are often made as sugar pellets to be placed under the tongue; they may also be in other forms, such as ointments, gels, drops, creams, and tablets. Treatments are "individualized" or tailored to each person—it's common for different people with the same condition to receive different treatments. There is very little to no valid scientific data to prove homeopathy to be effective for treating any specific condition. However, doctors and patients continue to recommend and use them successfully. I have personally used homeopathic preparations for the majority of my adult life and cannot deny the relief I have experienced as well as improvements I've seen in my patients. My personal philosophy is that no one should ever place their primary care in the hands of homeopathy. Instead it should be used as an adjunctive form of care for things such as relieving symptoms and/or removing toxins from the body.

6. **Pulsed Electromagnetic Therapy (PEMF)** – PEMFs address impaired chemistry and thus the function of cells—which in turn, improves health. PEMFs deliver beneficial, health-enhancing PEMFs and frequencies to the cells. Low frequency PEMFs of even the weakest strengths pass right through the body, penetrating every cell, tissue, organ, and even bone without being absorbed or altered! As they pass through, they stimulate most of the electrical and chemical processes in the tissues. Therapeutic PEMFs are specifically

designed to positively support cellular energy, resulting in better cellular health and function. PEMF has been recommended for a host of health problems. Scientific studies have shown its ability to reduce pain, inflammation, the effects of stress on the body, and platelet adhesion, improve energy, circulation, blood and tissue oxygenation, sleep quality, blood pressure and cholesterol levels, the uptake of nutrients, cellular detoxification and the ability to regenerate cells, balance the immune system and stimulate RNA and DNA, accelerate repair of bone and soft tissue, and relax muscles.[7]

FIX#4: Pain Stoppers

- Add more of the foods listed that elevate Nrf2 levels to your diet.

- Supplement with some or all of the compounds that were listed that raise Nrf2 levels.

- Start doing HIIT training to improve the mitochondrial system and raise Nrf2 levels.

- Eliminate all excitotoxins from the diet. Supplement with pregnenolone if you are currently, or have been previously consuming any excitotoxin foods.

- Identify any genetic predispositions to inherited disorders and avoid habits that promote them and develop health strategies that prevent them.

- Test for MTHFR mutations and supplement with an MTHFR formula if you test positive.

- Choose the STOP THE PAIN PROTOCOL from the Six to FIX Recovery Protocols that apply to you and continue for at least 90 days. If more than one apply, you can combine protocols or, you can choose one and start the others after each one is completed in succession.

- Consider some of the alternative practices listed if they are appropriate for your particular health issue.

1. Sulforaphane Improves Lipid Metabolism by Enhancing Mitochondrial Function and Biogenesis in vivo and vitro. Lei P1, Tian S1, Teng C1, Huang L1, Liu X1, Wang J2, Zhang Y3, Li B2, Shan Y1. Mol Nutr Food Res. 2018 Dec 22:e1800795. doi: 10.1002/mnfr.201800795. [Epub ahead of print].

2. The Role of Pregnenolone in Inflammatory Degenerative Brain Disease Ferri C1 and Fioranelli M1, 2* 1Marconi University, Rome, Italy 2University B.I.S. Group of institutions, Punjab Technical University, Punjab, India: Citation: Ferri C and Fioranelli M (2014) The Role of Pregnenolone in Inflammatory Degenerative Brain Disease. Interdiscip J Microinflammation 1:121. doi: 10.4172/2381-8727.1000121:Received date: November 23, 2014; Accepted date: December 04, 2014; Published date: December 06, 2014.

3. Overdoing Acetamenophen; Harvard Health Letter; Harvard publishing; Harvard Med School: published: Aug. 2009.

4. Ozone therapy: A clinical review A. M. Elvis and J. S. Ekta J. Nat Sci Biol Med. 2011 Jan-Jun 2(1):66-70.

5. Acupuncture for Chronic Pain Individual Patient Data Meta-analysis Andrew J. Vickers, DPhil; Angel M. Cronin, MS; Alexandra C. Maschino, BS; et. al: Oct 22, 2012.

6. Hahnemann, Samuel (1833). The homœopathic medical doctrine, or "Organon of the healing art." Dublin: W. F. Wakeman. pp. iii, 48–49.

7. Dr. Pawluk: Medical authority on Magnetic Field Therapy; drpawluk.com.

NEURAL REPROGRAMMING

CHAPTER TEN

Neural Reprogramming

Reestablish Neural
Balance and Tone

Balancing the brain. The brain and nervous system control the structure, function, and coordination of the entire body (see page four of *Gray's Anatomy* for details). There are about one hundred billion brain cells contained within the human brain. Electrical sparks called nerve impulses speed along neural pathways and are processed, directed, or redirected to help establish homeostasis in the body. If the communication is normal and uninterrupted, then the body has "normal" function. This is called a balanced central integrated state (C.I.S.)

If for any reason that system of communication gets interrupted, the C.I.S. becomes imbalanced and the body will experience some form of dysfunction. Dysfunction eventually produces symptoms, which can manifest in a multitude of presentations in which pain is present most of the time.

One of the most common symptoms experienced from nerve

interference is pain. Pain is the primary motivation that causes people to seek doctors for help. Having a good understanding about certain brain-based problems can prevent a lot of wasted time and money spent on unnecessary and unwarranted treatments. Most people would be shocked to know how many problems can be resolved just by balancing the brain and its pathways. Everything that is experienced in life is perceived in the brain or it doesn't exist in the reality of the person experiencing it. So, basically, from the standpoint of realization, if it doesn't happen in the brain, it doesn't happen in your world.

Pain is not experienced at the place where the symptom appears; instead it's experienced in the brain. Knee pain is not experienced in the knee any more than stomach pain is experienced in the stomach. If you don't believe me ask a scientist what happens if you damage the sensory centers in the brain that are connected to the knee and stomach. He would tell you that you would no longer be able to feel pain in the stomach or the knee. All pain is experienced in the brain. The brain simply receives and transmits the information presented to it. Brain balance is crucial for vibrant health, agility, and mobility. Balancing aberrant brain pathways can be the key to resolving chronic pain. When pain pathways continue to fire afferent pain responses repeatedly for long periods of time, they can become very efficient at reporting the pain. Chronic pain syndromes develop multiple nerve networks through the process called neuroplasticity. It can be quite difficult in some cases to initially override these efficient pathways. Often more aggressive maneuvers and treatments are used to break the chronic pain cycles so the pain network is less efficient. Consistent repetitive motions over a long period of time can be used to rebalance the neural deficits created from those destructive cycles. Repatterning the pathways with focused maneuvers can be extremely beneficial for those who have neurological issues that need to be corrected.

Balanced Brain, Balanced Body

Eye movements, hearing, vision, body movements, internal thoughts, facial expressions, touch, thermal changes, postural changes, etc., are just a few examples of the things that stimulate our brain. If someone is out of shape it's quite obvious that they cannot perform at their highest capacity. They can get to a point where they are so out of shape that they find it difficult to do even the most menial tasks. Think of what it would be like if someone had an out of shape brain. I think it would be safe to assume that it might not be able to keep up with some of the demands placed upon it. This should reveal itself more and more the longer the brain stays in this condition. What if the brain was exercised just like the body when it's out of shape. Doesn't it seem pretty obvious that it would be capable of doing a much better job of handling the daily demands and overall function would be noticeably improved? That's exactly what happens when the brain is balanced. When the condition of the brain improves the entire body reaps the benefit. Proper balance is achieved by proper training. Yes, the brain can be trained just like the muscles in your body. The more consistent the training, the better the outcome for the body. Everything works better when the brain is in balance. Mental clarity, alertness, improved sleeping habits, more energy, relief from pain, and enhanced sense of well-being can all be expected and more, once the brain has been trained and brought back into balance.

BALANCE TEST

Step 1- Stand straight in an erect posture with your feet together, hands at your side, and with your eyes closed for one full minute if you are able. (Have someone film your test so after you've done the program for a while you can monitor your improvements.)

a) Watch for leaning and/or falling toward any direction.

b) Observe the posture and check for shoulder and pelvis un-leveling. Notice if the head is turned and/or tilted. Look and see if one of the feet are rolled in or out and if the nose falls in the middle of the line formed between the feet.

c) Check to see if there's any trunk twisting or leaning.

d) Keep the eyes closed and stand on one foot and bend the other knee up waist high as if you were marching. Hold that position for fifteen seconds, then repeat and do the other side. No practicing or do-overs, the first try is the results that are recorded or else it's not a valid test. When you re-do it you are temporarily training the brain and it skews the results. This is not a test you want to cheat on because the only person you're cheating is yourself.

Step 2 - March in place with arms raising high over your head as you march, At the same time turn your head all the way to the left and then all the way to the right continuing back and forth leaving the eyes closed the entire time for 15 marches both sides. Check and see if you are still facing straight ahead; if you moved or deviated from where you stared, then you failed the test.

Step 3 - close your eyes and march in place while tucking your chin to your chest and then lean your head all the way back as if you were looking up and down for 15 times while marching. Then check to see if you moved or deviated from center. If you did then you failed the test.

All of these tests should show the head facing straight ahead, level, balanced, no movement of the body, and head over center. If you have any of these imbalances, you definitely should consider doing this program. Keep a record of the imbalances so you will have a baseline to compare them to. Recheck every couple of weeks and film and record your progress. If after doing the exercises consistently each day for a couple of weeks you don't see any improvement or if you get worse, you may want to be examined by a physician to rule out a different underlying cause. Send your success stories and pics into our website so we can post the before and afters and tell your story to help encourage others.

STOP THE PAIN "TRAIN THE BRAIN" Balance Exercise

❝ ...better brain = better you!"

The **TRAIN THE BRAIN balance exercise** consists of some very specific exercises that help engage areas of the brain that commonly get imbalanced. The eyes cause muscles along and around the spine to activate and relax depending upon the position and posturing of the head. When spinal biomechanics are altered in the body it affects the head position, which also causes the visual response to report differently to the brain. When the righting reflex is intact and the cerebellum is balanced bilaterally, it keeps the head centered. Therefore, the body's posture centers to that head position. Often when there's a functional curvature of the spine, it's caused from weakened brain pathways that are contributing to the poor posture. When the eye muscles are strengthened and balanced from precision training and repetitive motion, the result can produce improved postural integrity, better balance, increased agility, better focus, and improved overall performance. When brain pathways are continually and repetitively stimulated, they become more efficient. This can be all summed up with one statement, "**better brain = better you!**" Follow the instructions exactly the way they are explained and continue the process each day. Remember, continual repetitive motion is what regenerates brain pathways, so make the TRAIN THE BRAIN balance protocol a part of your daily routine and enjoy the benefits of getting your brain in shape.

EXERCISE 1: FOCAL FIXATION ACTIVATION

Take three index cards and draw a one-inch circle in the center of each one and color the inside of the circle with a marker. You can use a quarter as a template. Place one in the center of the wall and the others approximately eight to ten feet on either side so that they are in a straight horizontal line. Stand about ten feet behind the center circle lining up directly behind it. The two balance poses for this exercise will be performed from this position. Get in the balance pose one position. Stare at the spot on the center of the card for three seconds, then to the left spot for three seconds, then back to the center for three seconds. Then to the right spot for three seconds and back to the middle and keep repeating while holding the poses in perfect posture. Try to remain still without swaying or moving around, keeping your head straight ahead, moving only your eyes and not your head. Get in the balance pose two position and repeat the same exercise.

Each time you shift the eyes from spot to spot, move the eyes quickly to the next spot as if you were snapping the eyes into the next position.

Change back to balance pose one position and this time close your eyes, maintaining the pose for an audible fifteen second count (one thousand one, one thousand two, etc.).

Change back to balance pose two, close your eyes and repeat.

Go back to balance pose one and start all over again, repeating this sequence over and over until you've achieved the desired amount of sets.

Balance pose one: Stand on the right foot with the left knee bent and lifted waist high while pointing the fingers on the right hand toward the ceiling with your arm over your head (right arm straight up) and the left arm straight fibers pointing at the floor, as if you were marching.

Balance pose two: Repeat the same thing opposite side.

Do the exercise in each pose for one minute and then repeat on the other side.

Start out doing one set on each side working up to three sets on each side.

If you are a competitive athlete, work up to five or more sets on each side and increase the eyes closed time to one full minute while maintaining perfect posture in the pose.

To really make it challenging for those who are advanced, do a small hop with the eyes closed while in the poses and land keeping your eyes closed the entire time. Do 10 or more hops on each side.

EXERCISE 2: ACCOMMODATION ACTIVATION

Sit upright in a chair with an excellent posture. Put your arm straight out in front of you at eye level with the thumb in an upward position so that the eyes are looking level at the thumbnail and bring it as close to your nose as you can without losing focus. Focus on the details of your thumbnail for the count of three while at the same time tightening up your stomach muscles, and then relax. Pick a spot on the other side of the room directly behind the thumb (like a light switch or a small object on a counter, etc.). Focus your vision on the specific details of the object. Hold it for the audible count of three while tightening up the stomach muscles, then relax. Continue repeating this exercise alternating back and forth repeatedly about 20 times. You can work up to 50 times if you like.

EXERCISE 3: OCULAR ACTIVATION

Sit upright in a chair with an excellent posture. Put your head in a facing forward position keeping it level with the horizon and keep it from moving left or right during the exercise. Raise your eyes in an upward gaze until they can go no further and pick a spot on the ceiling to focus on (Make sure you keep your head from tilting back). Next, try harder to push the eyes even further upward creating a bit of a strain on the eyes and find a spot to focus on that maintains that strain for a count of three (tighten up the stomach muscles at the same time while staring at doing the eye focus). Repeat this same technique while looking down at the floor, looking left, looking right, looking up and to the right, looking down and to the left, looking up and to the left, and looking down and to the right. These eye positions are referred to as the fields of gaze. Repeat this exercise three to five times to complete one set. [*Reminder - you must keep the head level and completely still while engaging in this exercise.]

Balance and stabilization are two of the most important functions necessary for supporting and facilitating movement. The TRAIN THE BRAIN balance protocol is designed to establish stronger and more efficient neural pathways in order to better support the posture and allow for better balance and agility. Moving efficiently prevents unwanted wear and tear on the joints, muscles, and tissues, and prevents degeneration that can ultimately cause pain and discomfort. Building plasticity in weakened pathways takes repetitive and consistent movements performed over a period of time. At first you may not be able to tell if the exercises are helping, but stay committed and follow the protocol and in a few weeks and months the benefits should be obvious.

NRGenics®: It's All in Your Head!

The brain's primary function is survival. The second is to transmit and receive neurological impulses. Its function is dependent upon the constant availability of **fuel, oxygen (O2)**, and **activation**, i.e., You have to give it fuel to power it and provide activity to spark the energy to make it work. When the fuel, O2, and activation are increased, the brain cells become more stable and may grow as a result. This type of growth may be termed as **neural plasticity**. If they are decreased, the cell becomes less stable, and can atrophy and even perish, making it less able to handle any demand placed on it. The medical term for this process is called **transneural degeneration**. When brain cells are deprived of the sufficient amount of fuel and activation the area generally associated typically makes a shift towards cell death. This is another reason for the occurrence of brain degeneration.

The plasticity of neural pathways is dependent on a mechanism referred to as "**frequency of firing**"(FOF). The stronger the stimulus, the stronger the FOF. That simply means when you do an activity it sends an electrical impulse along the nerves all the way to the brain. The nerves are firing impulses into the brain. The more you increase the activity the more you increase the electrical impulses firing through the nerves into the brain. When specifically coordinated exercises are done in a particular sequence, the nerves fire the electrical impulses through the pathways in the brain and create a balance. The NRGenics® program does exactly that. It works toward balancing the left and right hemispheres of the brain by engaging muscle groups to fire in a specific sequence to have the brain reset the body's gain parameters and bring things back into balance. Think of all of the slips, trips, and falls you've had. How many times have you bumped your head or ran into something? Take a moment and think about all of the injuries you've had in your lifetime. These injuries cause damage which changes the way the nervous system fires the brain causing, in some cases, gross imbalances. Have you ever retrained those neural pathways back into a balanced state? If you haven't, why not start right now?

NEURAL REPROGRAMMING (NRG) is the process of reestablishing the function of nerve networks that have either been injured or destroyed from some sort of acute, traumatic, or chronic process. Sometimes the damage is caused from the accumulation of small injuries over a period of time. People do everything from bumping their heads, slipping and falling, being exposed to toxic substances, constantly exposed to electromagnetic waves, to having chronic inflammatory processes all of which damage the brain and nervous system. The accepted belief up until the year 2000 was that the central nervous system did not regenerate. That meant if you damaged brain or spinal cord it would be a permanent injury with no chance for a recovery. However, in the year 2000, two brilliant scientists, Kendell and Schwartz, won the Nobel prize for their discovery that the central nervous system can regenerate and have a chance for a recovery after its been damaged. The gist of the study was that they immobilized a cat's leg by putting a cast on it. They studied the corresponding brain connection and discovered that when the leg didn't move, the pathways became inactive and the brain began to atrophy and degenerate in that area. This actually proved the old adage, "If you don't use it, you'll lose it!" This finding itself was extraordinary but was only a glimpse of the promising reality that was about to be revealed. The most amazing part of the experiment was when they removed the cast and started continually exercising the cat's leg, not only did the leg muscles recover but so did the brain and the pathways connected to it. The term for this phenomenon is called "**NEURAL PLASTICITY.**" It's the formation and reformation of brain and its communication pathways. The takeaway message from this award-winning event is "**MOVEMENT HEALS!**" Patients ask me all of the time, "What can I do to start getting healthier?" The answer is simple: "MOVE" as much as you can and as long as you can without overdoing it. Start slowly and build up over time integrating as many body parts and as many different movements as possible. Activating the body to activate the brain is an exciting concept and the possibilities are endless. The stronger the brain the better the body can function. What a concept! The brain runs the body, and that means, "**It's all in your head!**"

This new concept rocked the world of neurology. This new discovery brought hope back to millions of people who, prior to, had no chance for recovery. The new science and treatment formats began to rapidly emerge and to this point have even included everything from stem cells to electrical implants. I actually attended an updated 350-hour diplomate in Functional Neurology program because I had to relearn and rethink the way I was conventionally trained. The experience broadened my horizons as a physician and challenged me on a professional and personal level, to develop protocols that could incorporate this new technology. After many years of development, the NRGenics® program has become a powerful tool to assist someone in attempting to balance nerve pathways and gain better balance and agility. The proverbial "couch potato" all the way up to the Olympic athlete level can utilize the program. The program and concept are simple to perform but the user establishes the intensity level. Precise, well-coordinated, specific repetitive movements at a steady pace cause nerve impulses to bombard the nervous system and brain causing pathways to be strengthened and even new pathways to be formed (NEUROPLASTICITY). The repetitive motions used are designed to provide better function, balance, and improved agility. It can be used in conjunction with other workouts and training programs but the **basic program** should be used to start the session and conclude it so the brain achieves balance while the muscles and tissues heal following the training. The basic program takes 10 to 15 minutes per session and is recommended three times a week minimum. That's a small commitment to make considering the amount of results that can be achieved.

Most who follow it quickly transition to doing it every day because they achieve significant results and feel much better as a result. The objective in doing the basic program is not to try to turn someone into a top level athlete but instead attempting to get everyone to "MOVE" in a way that science has already proven restores the balance in the brain and nervous system pathways. The basic program is actually the warmup and cooldown for the intermediate and advanced programs. The **intermediate program** is for those who enjoy a little more vigorous training using specific resistance coupled maneuvers along with HIIT for those who want the most results in the shortest amount of time. Then there is the **advanced program**. This is for the serious athlete who wants to have the kinetic advantage over other athletes while at the same time becoming nearly resilient to injuries. This program includes very intense multiple neurologically balanced coupled maneuvers done simultaneously that bring about fatigue at a very rapid rate. This allows for more intensity creating more power for increased endurance. The program concept and technique can be applied to any type of specialized sport and/or any type of athletic training.

For anyone who is interested in either of these programs, contact the website at drhannen.com for more info.

BASIC WORKOUT PROGRAM

Exercise 1: Cross crawl march (50 reps each side). March while staying in one spot with the knees raising parallel to the ground, arms straight, one pointed at the ceiling and one at the ground, alternating sides.

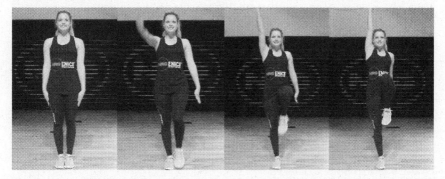

Exercise 2: Straight arm straight leg cross crawl march (50 reps each side)

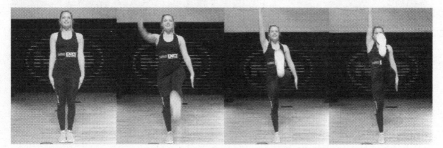

Exercise 3: Shoulder rolls (small first, medium next, and then large) forward and reverse (5 reps fingers down, 5 reps fingers up, with each step) total of four steps forward; then reverse the direction of arm rotation and repeat doing four steps backwards.

Small Rolls

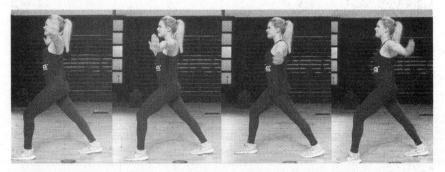

Medium Rolls

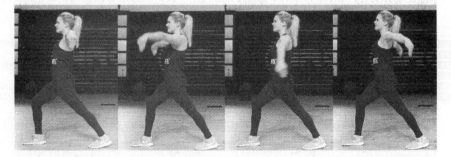

Large Rolls (hands in neutral position)

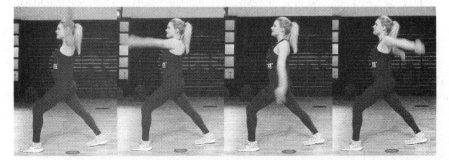

Exercise 4: Cross crawl lunge position stretch. Step out in a lunge position with the left arm extended up alongside of head and the right arm on position down behind you while slowly stretching, keeping the back leg straight to feel the stretch in the calf muscle. Hold the stretch pose for 10 seconds. Repeat on the other side.

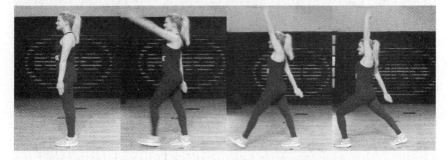

Exercise 5: Reverse cross crawl standing stretch balancing on one leg (hold for 15 seconds each side and do it twice)

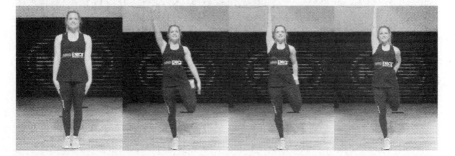

Exercise 6: Toe touches. Bend forward at the waist until you meet first resistance, hold for three seconds, then try to touch your toes for 20 seconds.

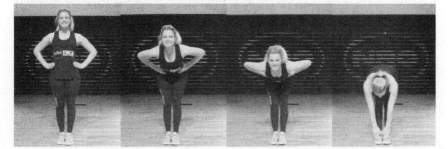

Exercise 7: Crossovers with wrist extension (bend forward until you meet first resistance, hold for 3 seconds then try to touch your toes for 20 seconds). Repeat on the other side.

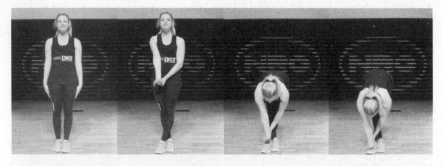

Exercise 8: Straddle stretch - spread legs apart as far as you can. Cross arms and lean forward letting your head and elbows hang toward the ground for 30 seconds.

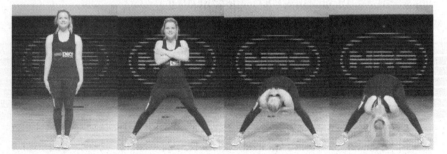

Exercise 9: Stand tall on the wall – this exercise is done immediately at the end of the workout. Place your back against a wall with the arms at your side (thumbs facing forward) and the back of the heels touching the wall as well. Press your entire body against the wall. Try to press the back of the head into the wall taking the head straight back (like a chicken picking corn) keeping the head level without looking up or tilting the head back. Hold the erect posture pressing the entire body against the wall for 3-5 minutes. When you walk away from the wall you should feel very upright and erect in your posture if you did it correctly.

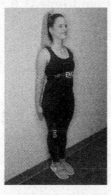

This exercise can also be used to assist in correcting poor posture when performed morning and night, daily. If you have any questions about the exercises, please feel free to contact us at drhannen.com.

NRGenics® Gives You Energy (NRG)

Take the "**BASIC BALANCE TEST**" and find out if you have any obvious balance issues. Grade yourself fairly and accurately so after you've done the program for a while you can retest and see the improvement. It's so exciting and even fun to literally watch your body improve so dramatically from just making some good choices. This program might not cure all of your problems but it can definitely be a huge step in the process of your recovery. Everyone can use some neural reprogramming and can benefit from its effects on the body. Enjoy your neural reprogramming sessions using the NRGenics® training program and start the journey down your road to recovery so you can STOP THE PAIN from stopping you.

Emotional Abuse (Emotional Gut)

There are millions of people worldwide who suffer with a condition called **irritable bowel syndrome (I.B.S.)**. It's a condition that consists of erratic bowel habits that can cause discomfort, pain, and even inconvenience. There was an interesting study[1] done that showed that the majority of the people studied who had been sexually abused, at some point in their life, would develop IBS. That doesn't mean if you have IBS that you were sexually abused. The study simply demonstrated that if someone had ever been sexually abused there is a high likelihood that they could develop IBS. There appears to be a strong connection between emotional trauma and the effects it can have on the digestive system and more specifically, the bowel. Many years ago I developed an entire Road To Recovery program. Individuals often go through the program and are able to sort out some of the thoughts and emotions that have been tormenting them for years. People need to be reminded that the abuse they experienced did not happen because of something they did wrong. It's quite common to find victims of abuse internalizing these horrific events to the point they convince themselves they are bad people, damaged goods, or worse yet , that something is wrong with them. I've been involved in all types of programs trying to find what brings benefit and what doesn't and I've come to the conclusion based on my own personal experience of nearly thirty years, that faith-based programs seem to bring the most dramatic, impactful, and lasting change compared to the others. One of the first steps in overcoming any hurtful or abusive situation is **forgiveness**. Holding on to the things from the past continues to tie you to that situation. The truth is the pain that comes from that situation cannot leave you until you release what ties you to it. The first and most important step is forgiveness. Forgive the person who caused the abuse. The reason you forgive someone is not because they deserve it, it's because it separates you from the event emotionally and allows the healing process to begin. People who have I.B.S., depression, and other problems associated with the trauma from abuse, have emotional brain pathways that negatively stimulate the body's nervous system all the way down deep within the gut. Thoughts and emotions can wreak havoc on the autonomic system producing stress and all kinds of unexplained symptoms. Emotions produce thoughts; thoughts produce conflict; conflict produces stress; stress produces symptoms, disorders, and even disease; these issues tend to drain the energy systems leaving them depleted, fatigued, suppressed and oppressed; this in turn causes more feelings of despair, hopelessness and helplessness which further traumatizes them emotionally; and the vicious cycle continues to repeat itself. Sometimes sufferers have these issues for years and the emotional ties become emotional knots that can take some time to untie. People who suffer from emotional pain and trauma quite often deal with chronic pain as well. I've treated certain patients over the years who have been diagnosed with fibromyalgia, chronic fatigue, and other painful conditions like these, who have been able to overcome their disorders as a result of getting their emotional issues resolved. Emotions are powerful stimulants to the nervous system and can be beneficial or detrimental depending on whether the emotion was positive or negative in nature. It's common for people dealing with fear to experience anxiety and stress. On the flip side, it's quite common for people who are at peace to experience feelings like that of euphoria along with a sound state of being. Emotions control the way we think, behave, and conduct our lives. They are the awareness of experience that ties us to a moment. Emotions control us. When our emotions are out of control, our lives can be affected on a lot of different levels. When people internalize their problems, that in itself becomes the problem. There are people out there who have stuffed their problems for years and as a result they are walking around in pain and suffering because the physical has now been affected by the emotional. In my book *Healing by Design*, I dedicated an entire section to beating depression. You may find it very useful if you are trying to overcome this condition. This book is more focused on the physical aspects of pain. It would require writing another entire book to cover all of the aspects of emotional causes of pain and suffering. However, one thing I have learned after this many years of experience, is that when you make your body and brain strong and healthy, your emotions usually follow.

FIX#5: Pain Stoppers

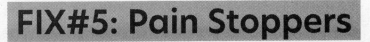

- Take the balance test and film it to document the results.

- Begin doing the **TRAIN THE BRAIN** balance exercises each and every day to help to strengthen those neural pathways.

- Engage in doing the **NRGenics® program** to assist your body in renewing and rebuilding the plasticity in the neural system that has aged over your lifetime. Neural reprogramming should be enjoyable and not a dread. It may seem a little tough at first, but as you continue it will get easier and easier and the rewards and benefits will far outweigh the brief struggle experienced while getting started.

- Honestly evaluate your emotional status and determine if you have any emotional baggage. Start out by forgiving the people in your past and release yourself from any toxic emotions. If needed, you can go online to drhannen.com and see if you might benefit from the **Road to Recovery program**.

1. Irritable Bowel Syndrome: Relationships with Abuse in Childhood; Randy A. Sansone, MD; Innov Clin Neurosci. 2015 May-Jun; 34-37.

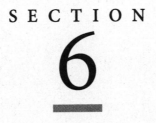

SECTION

6

SPIRITUAL ALIGNMENT

CHAPTER ELEVEN

Spiritual Alignment

Prayer and Fasting

In the Bible, the apostle Paul makes an insightful statement instructing to "Pray without ceasing!" Imagine how our health might improve if we all followed that advice every day. Most every religion known to man involves some form of meditation and prayer. Prayer is a way to spiritually align us. We consist of a three-part being of spirit, soul, and body. The body can be healed, the soul can be delivered, but the spirit needs to be aligned. If you align it with God, it will be like God. If you align it with other things, it will become like other things. Prayer is basically a direct connection and access to a higher spiritual power. If you pray to a higher power, then that power becomes available to you. Praying is simply becoming one with whatever power you are praying to. For example, millions of Christians have aligned themselves with Jesus Christ and as a result their spirits are renewed, allowing healing and restoration to take place in their lives. If you believe prayer doesn't work, then it probably won't work for you.

Please be watchful what you connect yourself to. When people have been in situations where they have suffered with pain and agony for years, they become desperate. When people become desperate they do desperate things. I personally know of many cases where people turned to other things instead of prayer. Those stories did not have a happy ending. Alcohol is not the answer. Drugs are not the answer. Opioid pain relievers are not the answer. Praying and having faith in the prayer you are praying because of the One you're praying to is the answer.

There is an invisible force that exists when someone prays a prayer of faith. There's some kind of exchange that takes place that cannot be measured in the natural realm. It exists only in the supernatural realm. It exists when God adds super to your natural. The Bible calls it "the prayer of faith" and declares, "**The prayer offered in faith will make the sick person well...**" (James 5:15, NIV). This apparently isn't just a belief. Science is now confirming it to be the truth. Even the scientists in the secular world have documented prayer promotes healing. Study after study, they show how the power of prayer and meditation can make the sick person well.

❝ Prayer is the most widespread alternative therapy in America today. ❞

According to scientists, prayer and meditation are not mere practices for someone of faith, but are a viable option to assist in improving the quality of health. Prayer and meditation have been found to produce a clinically significant reduction in resting as well as ambulatory blood pressure,[1] to reduce heart rate,[2] to result in cardiorespiratory synchronization,[3] to alter levels of melatonin and serotonin,[4] to boost the immune response,[5] to decrease the levels of reactive oxygen species (oxidation),[6] to reduce stress and promote positive mood states,[7] to reduce anxiety and pain and enhance self-esteem.[8]

Most everyone should be able to find 15 minutes for prayer and meditation each day to help their body reduce its levels of stress, inflammation, and oxidation. First Corinthians 12:9 combines faith and prayer under the category of gifts of healing. A gift is something that is free. Where else can you get daily treatments that remove these degenerative processes in an endless supply with no cost to the user without side effects? However, like any other treatment, you have to actually do it in order to receive the benefit. Prayer is the most widespread alternative therapy in America today. More than 85 percent of people confronting a major illness pray, according to a University of Rochester study presented June 6 at the American Society of Clinical Oncology meeting in New Orleans. That is far higher than taking herbs or pursuing other nontraditional healing modalities. And increasingly the evidence is that prayer works.

Intermittent Fasting

Recent research studies reveal another practice that increases Nrf2 levels in the body, which also lowers NF-kB levels lowering inflammation and oxidation. This is quite popular in many circles and has been used for thousands of years for everything from detoxing to purification. This practice is called intermittent fasting. When you fast for up to 14-hour intervals at a time, it is referred to as "**intermittent fasting**." Science has proven that intermittent fasting causes Nrf2 levels to improve which lowers NF-kappaB levels and puts the Hulk back in the cage, which significantly reduces the level of inflammation and oxidation in the body. According to the research, you should be fasting on a regular basis. When Jesus gave instructions to His disciples, He did not say, "If you fast" He said, "When you fast." While in a fasting state you block the harmful effects of inflammation and oxidation on the body. A good way to start is by not eating any food after 6:00 p.m. and do not eat again until around 10:00 the next morning. Break the fast with a protein and carb together There are some people that teach you should eat like a king in the morning, a queen at lunch, and a peasant at supper. That may work for some people, but personally and professionally, I do not feel this is the best approach.

Many years ago, I started polling people that appeared to be physically trim and healthy, which will be referred to as **Group 1**. I then polled the next group of individuals who seemed to always struggle with their weight and physically appeared overweight and out of shape, which I will refer to as **Group 2**. A lot of the individuals in Group 1 did not exercise regularly, yet they appeared to be trim and in shape. On the other hand, a lot of the people in Group 2 exercised regularly and intensely, yet appeared to be overweight and out of shape. This was quite confusing at first, and the outcome may lead many to think that those in Group 2 must have some genetic predisposition that causes them to struggle with weight issues. There are many people out there today who actually embrace that mind-set. However, what I found out in the next part of this investigation was quite astounding and has been a life-changing discovery for those I have shared the information with. The apparent difference between Group 1 and Group 2 was that those in Group 1 did not eat breakfast. That means that every day they were doing intermittent fasting and their bodies were responding accordingly. When I discovered this phenomenon, I began sharing the information with the people in Group 2. You can probably predict what happened next. Yes, the people in Group 2 who stopped eating breakfast began to lose weight and even reported that they felt better. Since that time I have been able to share this information with countless people and many have reported back an immediate shift in metabolism. I have lost count of the number of patients presenting in my office who have tried multiple diets, supplements, exercise programs, and even prescription medications, and still struggle with their metabolism. Directing them to start doing something as simple as intermittent fasting has proven to be a game-changer for many of those who followed the recommendation. Fasting also allows the body to detoxify itself, ridding the body of toxic substances that can damage cells and lead to sickness, disease, and yes, even pain and suffering. Just like prayer, intermittent fasting should be part of your daily life and not just an event. When combined with prayer and meditation, the results can be astounding.

The thing to remember is that not only did the patients' metabolisms improve, but they claimed that they felt better as well. Looking and feeling better can sometimes be just a couple of decisions away. Intermittent fasting, prayer, and meditation are simple lifestyle choices you can make without having to spend money or purchase some product or device. Go ahead and start today, and do it every day so you will have the right tools working for you so you can look and feel better and STOP THE PAIN.

Practically every civilized culture throughout history has included fasting in one form or another in order to cleanse the body in an attempt to prevent and even eliminate sickness and disease. From a scientific standpoint the research is pretty solid. However, there is also a spiritual component that most every religion also embraces as well, that seems to bring about a spiritual clarity for those who participate in the fast. From metaphysical centering to balancing the body's chakras, new agers have discovered the value of scriptural truths. Whether these invisible energy systems exist or not is really not the topic, the truth is that we all seem to agree that the power of fasting is validated by centuries of repeated use. For Christians, the Bible records the use of the combination of prayer and fasting, especially for those who have toxic souls. In one particular account Jesus told His disciples the reason they were powerless to cast out a demon was because they were not following this important practice. Most everyone who is struggling spiritually can benefit from combining prayer and fasting. It's so much easier to hear and see with spiritual clarity when the emotional and spiritual garbage is removed from our present situations.

The same way we nourish our bodies with food is the same way we nourish our spirit: we have to feed it. The Holy Scriptures serve as the appetizing fresh, healthy, and fortifying nutrition for the soul and spirit. The same goes for prayer and fasting. Just as the combination of these two strategies cleanse the body, so it is with the soul and spirit as well. Out with the old (the trash from the past) and in with the new (the fresh revelation for your future). The apostle Paul defines the "complete being" so perfectly when he describes it as the whole spirit, whole soul, and whole body. All three parts need to be addressed in order to achieve complete wholeness. It's easy to get caught up in tending to your favorite part while the other parts lag behind and become unhealthy.

A good example of this is many of the people serving in the field of ministry. Often pastors who spend most of their time tending to others often forget to take the time to tend to their own needs. I personally know of many great pastors who are spiritually powerful, yet are beat up in their spirits and out of sorts in their bodies. Their spirits are willing but their flesh is weak. If you find yourself relating to the subject matter somewhere in this discussion, it may be a really good idea to go ahead and make a decision right now. How do you want to see yourself in the future? You are the one who holds the key to unlocking the potential inside of you to be the best you that you can be. Don't squander this opportunity. It should be quite obvious at this point that you are not reading this by accident. There is a real God and He cares about you enough to show you what to do in order to improve your present condition. Spirit, soul, and body has to be the focus for complete and total healing in order for you to reach your full potential. Prayer and fasting combined with making the changes that are revealed in this book could be the very thing that will be the turning point in your life that is necessary in order for you to STOP THE PAIN.

The sixth and final protocol will focus on repairing, regenerating, restoring, and reprogramming the brain and neural systems. This protocol should be utilized at the same time you are fixing the other five things that need fixed. It requires activity which promotes activation of the neural pathways. The only way this will be productive is if you do it consistently and repetitively and stay committed. Do it exactly as recommended and try not to do your version of the exercises. Follow the instructions through the entire book so you can FIX THE SIX and STOP THE PAIN.

6. NEURAL RECOVERY PROTOCOL

a)   Begin by taking the balance test and record your results. This is a good way to monitor your progress.

b)   Begin the **NRGenics™ program** and find the pace that works for your level of fitness. Continue to progress until you can do it without stopping at a steady, brisk pace.

c)   Do the **Four for the Core** exercises three or more times per week. Strengthening the core is essential for maintaining the integrity of the musculoskeletal and neural systems.

d)   Make intermittent fasting and prayer a part of your daily routine to assist with lowering inflammation and improving the healing process.

e)   Incorporate HIIT training into your exercise routines like riding a bicycle, running/jogging, swimming, jumping jacks, workouts, etc. If you are doing the NRGenics™ program at the intermediate or advanced level, the HIIT training has already been incorporated.

FIX#6: Pain Stoppers

● Pray and meditate for a minimum of fifteen minutes at least a couple of times each day. Find a quiet secluded or private place when you do so the things around you don't distract you.

● Start doing intermittent fasting each day and feel the improvement. Sometimes when you fast the body can release toxins giving you symptoms like a cold or the flu. Make sure you drink plenty of water and if necessary, break the fast until the symptoms subside. If you are diabetic, have blood sugar issues, are taking prescription medications, or have any other health-related risks, always consult your physician before engaging in any type of fast.

● Take all of the information you've received from this book and utilize the strategies that apply to your situation or circumstance. Many of the recommendations have no cost associated with them whatsoever, so there is something for everyone. The most important thing is to do something and to do it now.

1. Prayer and healing: A medical and scientific perspective on randomized controlled trials. Indian J psychiatry. 2009 Oct-Dec;51(4):247-253.

Anderson JW, Lou C, Kryscio R.J. Blood pressure response to transcendent all meditation: A meta-analysis, Am J Hypertensive. 2008;21:310-6 [PubMed].

2. Solberg E E, Ekeberg O, Holen A, Ingier F, Sandvik, Standal Pa, et. al. Hemodynamic changes during long meditation. Appl Psycophysical Biofeedback.2004;29:213-21 [PubMed].

3. Cysarz D, Blssing A. Cardiorespiratory synchronization during Zen Meditation. Eur J Appl Physiol. 2005;95:88-95.[PubMed].

4. Solberg E E, Holen A, Ekeberg O,Osterud B Halversen R.,Sandvik.,The effects of long-term meditation on plasma melatonin and blood serotonin.

5. Davidson RJ, Kabat-Zinn J. Schumacher J,,Rosenkranz M, Muller D , Santorelli SF. Alterations in brain and immune function produced on mindfulness meditation.

6. Van Wiik EP, Ludtke R, Van Wiik R, Different Al Effects of relaxation techniques on ultra weak photon emission.

7. Jan S, Shapiro S L, Swanick S, Roesch SC, Mills P.J., Bell I. A randomized controlled trial of mindfulness meditation verses relaxation training: Effects on Distress, Positive States of Mind, rumination, and distraction, Ann Behav Med. 2007;33:11-21. [PubMed].

8. Bonadonna R. Meditations impact on Chronic Illness. Holistic Nurs Practice. 2003;17:309-19. [PubMed].

In Conclusion

Final thoughts

Chronic pain and suffering can be overwhelming at times. It can leave you feeling helpless and hopeless. There is nothing more frustrating than going from doctor to doctor, specialist to specialist, clinic to clinic, or having test after test, and procedure after procedure, and still no one can find out what's causing the problem.

The sole purpose of this book is to better educate you so you can better understand where pain comes from, what causes it, and how to get rid of it. Once you understand the mechanisms that cause the pain, you start making the changes that need to occur in order to get rid of it.

Remember, the goal is not to cover it up, but instead get to the root cause. This information is to educate you so you can make informed choices when it comes time to make decisions about your health so you can STOP THE PAIN. If after completing it you still have questions, you may need to go back and read it again.

I personally recommend that while reading it if you see things that apply to you, highlight those areas so you can go back later and find them so you can start correcting them. Use the quick reviews of **pain stoppers** at the end of each chapter to remind you what to do to stay on track.

Order the protocols and get started while you're motivated, so you can start feeling better. Make sure you do the exercises recommended and stay consistent and committed. Do it right away before you get busy and fall back into a rut.

The **STOP THE PAIN** and the **SIX TO FIX DVD** series are also available and allows you the convenience of getting private instruction on some of these same topics. Our website is also dedicated to staying on the cutting edge of research and the newest scientific breakthroughs to keep you informed about your health. It's such a privilege to serve you in this capacity and to know that you have been given the tools you need to regain control of your health.

My prayers are with all of you as you get back on the road to recovery, and I'm believing that you are going to achieve great success and finally STOP THE PAIN.

Remember, "Health is a choice, choose life"!

Please feel free to contact us
if you have any further questions:

WEBSITE:
drhannen.com

Hannen Health Systems
707 Boll Weevil Circle
Enterprise, AL 36330
1(866) 362-7297
info@hannenhealth.com